STRUNG

OUT

STRUNG OUT

One Last Hit
and Other Lies that
Nearly Killed Me

A MEMOIR

Erin Khar

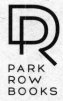

PARK
ROW
BOOKS

PARK
ROW
BOOKS™

Recycling programs
for this product may
not exist in your area.

ISBN-13: 978-0-7783-0973-4

Strung Out: One Last Hit and Other Lies That Nearly Killed Me

This edition published by arrangement with Harlequin Books S.A.

Park Row Books
22 Adelaide St. West, 40th Floor
Toronto, Ontario M5H 4E3, Canada
ParkRowBooks.com
BookClubbish.com

Printed in U.S.A.

For all those who didn't make it, who left too soon.
You are missed. You are loved.

Author's Note

Most names and identifying characteristics have been changed
to protect identities. Dialogue and order of events have been
reconstructed according to my memory, with the help of journals,
letters and conversations with those who were there. I have taken
great care to present the truth as I remember it.

STRUNG OUT

OUT

INTRODUCTION
Going to Get the Girl

What can be said of a thirteen-year-old girl's pain? What leads her onto the path of heroin?

Sometimes a girl moves through the crucibles of girlhood toward womanhood without realizing she's collecting pain all over her body, inside and out. What then shall be the language, the mode of self-expression in a world fast erasing her experience under the cover story of "woman"?

A girl could wake up one day with an unfillable hole in her heart and an unquenchable desire shooting out of her body.

I don't think individuals who are in pain are broken.

I think the world we're supposed to live in is broken, and that brokenness is too often reflected in our bodies. But we might be the ones who can help the world to heal. We have the skill set since we've been to the edges. We are the ones who are able to see more than one story at a time.

Erin Khar has written a resilience narrative, to be sure. *Strung Out* is the story of her addiction and subsequent recovery, but it is also the story of what was underneath that, what led to her addiction in the first place—and so the book pulls away from other recovery narratives because it is also something else: a resistance narrative.

Erin's story illuminates how the body of a girl and a woman is used by culture—sometimes used up or abused or used to death—and how sometimes that same woman might yet resist the debilitating impact of her culture by embarking on a rescue mission. Erin found the strength not only to survive, but also to resist what her culture was feeding her: *You are an attractive object. Your pain isn't real. You should stay quiet with your grief. Smile more. You should make your anger pretty and soft.* Her form of resistance was survival, from one of the most addictive drugs, yes, but moreover, from a society that doesn't value the body of a girl.

You could say *Strung Out* is a heart anthem, a song about how it is possible to bring yourself back to life even when you've got one foot, leg, half a body inside the mouth of death. By learning to tell the different stories inside her body, Erin released herself from the kind of shame that causes someone to self-destruct.

Addiction is a motherfucker. I'm not speaking lightly when I say that. I'm not referencing some trite, clichéd story about a tragic downfall and a miraculous recovery. No, I actually believe the simplicity of that cover story contributes to more pain and suffering, relapses and feelings of self-worthlessness if a person doesn't "fit" that specific narrative. Although I don't identify any longer with the word *addict*, which is the medicalized term for those of us who suffer in the ways that we do, I am a card-carrying member. The thing is, this tendency is lifelong. What we have has been historically stigmatized and remains so, and is often described as weakness, a personal failing. What we have comes and goes over the course of a lifetime, latent or triggered by God knows what's next. I am fifty-six, so I know a bit about how the boomerang works. Telling the story requires turning back on your own life and having a good, hard look, yes, but it also requires learning how to *see* differently. Some of the stories we are carrying inside us are contradictory, terrifying, ugly even.

How can you learn to truly see the self that did not want to feel anything? The self that moved deathward since life hurt too much? The self that felt emptied of worth? The self that created a cover being through drugs to get through existence—"that's the thing about grief—sometimes it's so sharp, you feel fearless"? And how can you learn to see her with compassion and kindness?

You go back and get your girl, that's how, which is what Erin Khar does in *Strung Out*. You retrieve your body's stories. You take them back from a culture, from families, from institutions, and from individuals who tried to write stories across your body, one line at a time.

And if you are lucky, then you invent how to *thrive* in the face of all the destruction.

Erin saved her own life. She made her way back to love and art and desire and life and motherhood and writing and thriving by letting go of one story of self and then taking the Big Risk of opening up to the world, the Big Risk of reaching for connection, the Big Risk of choosing self-expression over self-destruction, the Big Risk of letting all of her stories exist.

It doesn't matter how those of us who suffer achieve the ability to stay alive, to love, to thrive. There are so many ways to stay alive, and all of them are beautiful. Even those we have loved who found they could not keep going help the rest of us remember to breathe to honor them. Erin's story is one way to learn how to look back at your own life and learn to *see* a self worth saving. She was beautiful even inside her pain, even inside her decade-long opioid addiction, even inside her mistakes and grief.

Her beauty is her ability to share this story.

You have a beautiful life in your hands.

Lidia Yuknavitch

PROLOGUE

October 2015

"Mom, did you ever do drugs?"

The words of my twelve-year-old son, Atticus, lingered in the space between us. A car horn from the busy street outside could be heard from our fourth-floor apartment in Greenwich Village, punctuating the moment. Parts of myself, other selves, past selves, collided headlong into who I'd become—a mother, a wife, a writer, an advice columnist.

At that moment, I wanted time to stop. I wanted Atticus to remain too young to understand the perils of drug addiction. I know how drug use can obliterate a life; I didn't want any part of it to touch him. I wanted to protect him from the harsh realities of the opioid crisis that is ravaging our country. But this impulse to look away, to avoid confronting the opioid crisis and pretend it's not happening, is the very thing that keeps us in danger. How can we recover as families, as a nation, and create a healthier space for our children if we don't talk about it? We must be willing to share our experiences and be willing to examine the opioid crisis from all angles, even the angles that hit close to home.

The fact is every eleven minutes an American dies of drug overdose. Overdoses are the leading cause of death in this country for people under fifty-five.[1]

A lot has been reported about the role of the pharmaceutical industry in the opioid crisis. And undoubtedly, the proliferation of drugs like oxycodone flooding the market via doctors has created a whole new generation of opiate users who might not have found their way to addiction otherwise. That's not the whole story. Not everyone who gets a prescription for opioid painkillers becomes addicted, and not everyone starts with pills.

But over two million Americans are currently struggling with opiate addiction and nearly 20 percent of them are young adults. Even more staggering, use among young women is up, and the incidence of young pregnant women using opioids has increased by as much as 600 percent in some areas over a ten-year period.[2]

To say we have an opioid crisis is an understatement. You can't go a day, let alone a week, without the opioid epidemic infiltrating the news cycle.

And yet, so many people ask why anyone would do drugs in the first place.

The simplest answer is emotional pain. We live in a time in this country when everything moves so fast, when we are confronted by an altered view of other people's realities through social media, the social and political climate is divisive, and the guarantee of creating better lives for ourselves than our parents' generation has all but disappeared.

Our approach to mental health care is broken. Free and subsidized services are limited at best. The people who are most at

---

1 Josh Katz and Margot Sanger-Katz, "'The Numbers Are So Staggering.' Overdose Deaths Set a Record Last Year," *New York Times*, November 29, 2018, https://www.nytimes.com/interactive/2018/11/29/upshot/fentanyl-drug-overdose-deaths.html

2 Jennifer Egan, "Children of the Opioid Epidemic," *New York Times Magazine*, May 9, 2018, https://www.nytimes.com/2018/05/09/magazine/children-of-the-opioid-epidemic.html

risk—those in poor and marginalized communities—have financial and social barriers to accessing help.

The American ethos of putting your nose to the grindstone and persevering does a great disservice to our mental and emotional health. When you can't get out of bed in the morning, when you have no self-worth left, when you've had childhood trauma, when you suffer from any form of PTSD, the option of pulling yourself up by the bootstraps and overcoming addiction or other mental health issues is not possible. And that's not a moral failing.

The stigma associated with opioids, with heroin, with "being a junkie," prevents people from reaching out. And that stigma is killing us. Americans are stuck in a spiral of shame, and that shame drives the vicious cycle of relapse that many drug users get caught in.

The only way to break through that shame is by talking about it. It is terrifying to admit that you need help, to admit that you are addicted. This is especially true when it comes to heroin. Heroin use conjures up the gruesome images we see reported. Even among people who experiment with drugs, who drink and smoke pot and try cocaine, heroin represents some moral boundary—one that is reinforced by media. Those who cross that boundary, who "choose" to use heroin, are marked with shame.

Shame is a gatekeeper that prevents people from seeking help. Stigma is bred from that shame.

That stigma has killed so many. That stigma almost killed me.

I turned toward the television. Atticus had been half watching the news. A successful female dermatologist from Long Island had been found dead here in New York City, presumably from a drug overdose. She was married, had kids, seemed to have it all. The reporter speculated on the double life she led.

From my chair across the living room, I didn't look up from my book, ignoring the question that hung in the air like a balloon that was quickly deflating.

"Mom?"

"What was that, honey?"

"Did you ever do drugs?"

I paused again, suspended in the moment, making a quick mental inventory of how to answer. The truth is I did do drugs, a lot of drugs. I used heroin off and on from the age of thirteen until I got pregnant with Atticus at age twenty-eight. I never got into pot or alcohol. I'd needed something to take me further away. I took Valium and Vicodin, I dropped acid and took X and mushrooms, I smoked crack, shot the animal tranquilizer ketamine, and snorted the occasional line of crystal meth, but I always came back to heroin. I wasn't fucking around; I craved unconsciousness, but I wasn't about to tell my twelve-year-old son that. Not yet.

"That's a complicated question. You know, alcohol's a drug."

I tried not to visibly cringe at my own deflection at my son's question. Confusion spread across his face, between his freckles. He looks so much like me, except for the freckles, but we're so very different.

"Why do people take drugs?" he asked.

The first time I used, I took a pill. It was a Darvocet, an opiate. I stole it from my mother's medicine cabinet. The bottle was expired, with my grandmother's name on the label. I was eight.

"Well, people take drugs for different reasons. Sometimes, they try drugs because a friend talks them into it, or they are trying to escape something in their life. But drugs never help anything. They usually make things a lot worse."

I did not tell him that, in some ways, the drugs were once what kept me alive.

He squinted, scrunched his nose, clearly thinking about what I'd just said, licking his lips the way he does when he's concentrating. "I don't understand why someone would take drugs," he said definitively and walked out of the room.

A wave of nausea started at the top of my head, rippled down, anchoring itself in my stomach. Nausea was nothing new. Vaguely nauseous was homeostasis for me when I struggled with addiction. I put down my book and followed him. I saw my reflection in the hallway mirror. I was a healthy, happily remarried mother and writer. I was not the desperate and broken twenty-something, frighteningly thin and green all the time, the one who was married to his father for all the wrong reasons, the one who was constantly chasing an exit, any exit.

I stood at Atticus's open bedroom door. He was lying down on his bed with his iPhone in his hands, watching a video on YouTube. His bangs were getting too long, and he kept pushing the straight brown strands of hair aside. He looked just like he did when he was a baby, just like he did in the 3-D ultrasound photo I have, head to the side, one arm up, his hand in a fist against the cheek of his round face. But he was not a baby. He was in those awkward years between childhood and early adulthood, the years that demanded the conversations that I, as a mother, wanted to have with him, wish someone had had with me, but I was petrified. I didn't want to shatter his image of me. If he knew what I'd done, who I'd been, would he still respect me, still love me? Could I still be the mother I'd always been? Aren't you supposed to protect your children? Atticus was only a year younger than I was when I first started using heroin.

I knew I must have been doing something right because he didn't understand the impulse to use drugs. He thought they were stupid. He wasn't searching for a way out the way I had. We'd talked about it when we watched reruns of my all-time favorite show—*Beverly Hills, 90210*—together. He'd asked me questions—when David stayed up for days on end doing crystal meth, when Dylan smoked heroin and crashed his car, and when Kelly went on a cocaine binge with her boyfriend and landed in rehab. He had a concept of the consequences, but he didn't grasp the reasons. Until now, he'd never considered the possibility that I might have done drugs. And now this question.

How could I explain it to him? Would he understand? I thought about what I could impart by telling him—or telling someone who may be struggling with opioid addiction—my story. I wanted him to know that drug use doesn't look the same across race, class, and other privileges, but that it stems from a primal place of want and loneliness. I hoped that when the time came I would be successful in communicating a story of experience, strength, and hope, one that might make a difference.

CHAPTER 1
Thirteen
November 1986

Alone, in front of the stables where I kept my horse, I waited for Ted. I paced and then stopped, planting my feet beneath me, willing my body to stay still. I had changed out of my riding clothes, but traces of sweat collected in the creases of my body. My hair smelled like hay.

He pulled up in his dad's white Mercedes 560SL with the top down, his golden hair perfectly tousled. My hand on the door handle, electricity coursed through me. *He's too good-looking*, I thought. As I got in the car, he pulled me toward him by the back of my neck for our first kiss. I had just turned thirteen. He thought I was fifteen.

I'd met Ted and his cousin Sam earlier that year on a spring ski trip in Mammoth. I'd given him my phone number and we'd talked a few times. I'd gone to a party they'd invited me to a few months earlier and had since hung out with the two of them a couple of times. But now Ted and I were going out on a date—a real date—just the two of us. It was my first one, unless you counted the boys I'd gone to dances with or kissed at pool parties. This felt different.

We sped along Forest Lawn Drive, flanked by the cemetery on one side and the empty basin of the Los Angeles River and the Warner Brothers lot on the other, in the crisp November air. My long brown hair whipped around my neck like a collar. I could barely hear "Panic" by The Smiths over the sound of the car's engine, the rushing air, and the sound of my heart beating in my ears. I shut my eyes and reminded myself to breathe. The car turned down Barham, past the Hollywood Bowl, heading west on Franklin, and farther west on Sunset, and I could feel myself turning—away from who I'd been, pulled toward some possibility, some future I couldn't identify.

Ted lived in the Trousdale Estates, north of Sunset, overlooking Beverly Hills. We pulled into a long, immaculate driveway lined with tall, perfectly trimmed boxwood hedges and arrived in front of an imposing white, modern house. It was so different from mine. I lived with my mom in an eclectic Spanish house in a canyon, one that felt lived-in and heavy with the history of its occupants. Ted's parents were still married; he had an older brother, who was in college. My parents were divorced. But we were both marked by a specific type of absence, and I could feel it in the white walls in front of us. His house was a blank slate.

We walked through a humongous front door into the dark foyer. He flipped the lights on, walking ahead of me, and I followed, taking in all the white space. As we headed to the sunken living room, I looked through a wall of glass out to a shimmering pool that was all lit up.

"We can swim later if you want. It's heated."

I smiled in response. It wasn't the size of his house I found intimidating; it was its austerity, its angles and hard surfaces, cut like a diamond. Each and every light was perfectly placed to make the house glow.

"Do you want something to drink? A Coke? Water?" he asked.

"Sure. A Coke?"

He left the room, and I hated that I'd answered him like I was asking a question, like I was asking permission. I felt anxious about spilling my Coke on the couch or, worse, that some imperfection of mine would spill out, sullying all that white.

"Have you ever been surfing?" he asked, balancing two glasses and a bottle of Coke.

"No, actually, no."

As he continued to talk about surfing, I began to tune out, waiting for the next turn, a turn I couldn't identify but I felt was coming. Tuning out was what I did when I was anxious, when I sensed there was something happening in social situations beyond my control. I'd been doing it since I was in preschool. *Shut your eyes, hold your breath, count, leave, leave, leave.* By thirteen, I could do it and still pretend to be there.

We talked about The Velvet Underground and Rimbaud and Fassbinder films.

"Do you ever read *Details*?" I asked. "I have a subscription. I was reading this article about Warhol and The Velvet Underground, and, you know, they were really like an art project for him. But then they became something so much more. Are you into art? Basquiat is pretty interesting."

God, Erin, just shut up.

I worried that I was talking too much. I told him a dumb knock-knock joke, and he touched my face with his hand. He brushed my knee, and my leg erupted in goose bumps.

"Are you cold?"

"No, I'm okay."

"I like your skirt," he said, running his hand under the hem, resting it on my thigh.

"Thanks."

Ten days earlier, on my thirteenth birthday, my mom took me shopping. She bought me this short plaid skirt, with a large safety pin closure, in the weird mall that had just opened up in downtown Los Angeles. My mom, tall and blonde and underweight, leaned against the door frame of the dressing room.

She'd been going through a rough patch with her boyfriend. And by going through, I mean falling apart at the joints, unable to accept the inevitable demise of their relationship. The guy, a total prick, told her he didn't know if he could be with someone who already had a child. He was tall and blond and lean, like her. I was tall and lean but dark and looked like my father, and my mom's boyfriend hated me for it. Or I assumed he hated me for it. I didn't care what the real reason was because I hated him, too. It was the only thing we could agree on.

"You don't think it's too short?" she asked, moving toward me in the dressing room mirror with a concerned look on her face.

"NO, Mom."

I'd grown six inches in the past year, landing right around five-eight, taller than most of my eighth-grade classmates, definitely taller than the guys. I looked in the mirror and wondered if she was right. *Am I too tall now?* I felt too tall. I decided I didn't care.

That night, during my birthday dinner, my mom didn't eat, and I worked hard to fill the silence with insubstantial chatter. It was what I did best. With each passing day that her asshole boyfriend avoided her, I watched as my mother shrank in literal and physical stature. Watching her cede parts of herself, I felt a strong desire to harm myself.

I had struggled with the urge to kill myself—to cut myself out of my own skin—for many years. I remember at four and five and six, thinking I could just jump out the window; I could just get a knife and cut myself away. Whenever it got that I was feeling too much, that I didn't have enough body to contain everything humming under my skin, I faced that compulsion to annihilate myself—to stop and finally be still.

When I was eight, after my parents had separated, I *needed* to do something about it. My dad had moved out and my mother drifted from room to room in our old Spanish house with a weightlessness that I could tell threatened to take her away completely. I remember sitting in my room, on my brass bed, on a Saturday, picking at a scab on my knee. My mom was on the phone, upset—her voice muffled and far away. A panic spread across my chest, filling my body with heat, trapping me.

I ran to the bathroom and locked the door. As I reminded myself to breathe, some instinct led me to the medicine cabinet. I removed the Band-Aids and dental floss and the brown bottle of Betadine. I shook the bottle of Tylenol and held it for a moment. *I could take the whole bottle.* I had tried it once before, but I didn't take enough—my parents didn't even know I'd done it.

I saw a golden-brown pill bottle on the top shelf, next to the Pepto-Bismol. I held it in my hand, looking at the large red pills inside. It was Darvocet, my grandmother's name on the label; it was expired. May Cause Drowsiness or Dizziness, it read, next to the drawing of a man with droopy eyes and bubbles around his head. *Yes.* A voice inside that wanted to stop hurting urged me forward. I took a pill and put it in my mouth, gagging it down with gulps of water from the faucet.

Back in my room, I pulled *The World according to Garp* out from underneath my pillow and read. It was one of many books I snatched from the shelves in the den when I couldn't sleep. After a little while, the heat in my body was replaced by the lightness of little bubbles, and I remembered the label on the pill bottle. I felt like I might just float right out of my body. It was the exit I desperately wanted. That's when I started looking for pill bottles in medicine cabinets—at friends' and family members' houses—and when I'd feel that heat, when the need to cut myself out of my own skin became too much, I'd take a pill that came from a bottle with a warning label.

To avoid that empty feeling and to cover up sneaking pills,

I pushed myself forward, with straight As and horseback riding and cheerleading and volleyball, and filled my days with lots of friends and lots of chatter. *If I just shine bright enough, no one will notice anything.* But as the week following my thirteenth birthday wore on, I felt parts of me crumple and stay crumpled, like a collapsing star—dead, unable to reignite. And I did want to shine. I wanted to be told I was smart and special and good. I wanted proof—external, tangible proof—that I wasn't broken, that I was deserving of love. My spirit was at war with the ways I was coping. I wanted to be seen as desperately as I needed to hide.

Ted looked at me, narrowing his feline green eyes, and it made my stomach drop, made the crumpled parts of me bloom. He leaned in and kissed me, and I felt weightless. But underneath that weightlessness, some old wound pierced through, and it scared me. Unable to identify what it was or why Ted's hand resting on the side of my neck both thrilled and sickened me, I did my best to ignore it, whatever it was, letting it bang around and echo in some far-off edge of my memory.

"Let's go listen to music in my room," he said.

He didn't wait for me to answer and led me down a long hallway, one wall taken up by a large window, the city lights twinkling below. I sat on his bed, as he put on a Siouxsie and the Banshees record. He stood in front of me and said, "God, you're beautiful."

Am I? I wondered if he thought my hair smelled like hay. He pulled me up, and we stood in his room, kissing. I loved that he was taller than me, that he had strong arms, strong hands, that it felt like he could crush me. But I sensed myself sinking, and I needed—something. I needed something to push away the heat that filled my body and the voice that said, *You're broken and ugly and crazy and he'll find out and hate you.*

"Can I use your bathroom?" I asked.

He pulled me in, kissed me, and without saying anything led me, pushing me forward by my shoulders, to his bathroom. I closed the door behind me and took a deep, shaky breath. Like the rest of the house, the bathroom was white and pristine, out-fitted with marble and too many mirrors. It didn't look or feel like the bathroom of a sixteen-year-old guy. The mirrors came at me from every direction; I looked at myself and wondered what it was he saw. *You are not beautiful.*

I didn't have to use the bathroom; I flushed the toilet so it wouldn't seem weird, then turned on the faucet and let the water run. I put my fingers underneath and let the cool water trickle through the spaces in between. I opened the medicine cabinet and scanned the shelves for prescription bottles. There were none. My ears got hot, and I dabbed some water on them before shutting off the faucet.

"Do you want anything else to drink? A real drink?" he asked when I was back in his room.

"No, that's okay." *But I did want something.* "Do you have any Valium or Vicodin?"

He seemed surprised. He paused for a minute, then sat up. "Have you ever done heroin?"

"No."

"It's way better than pills."

"Do you have some?" I asked.

"Yeah."

"Okay."

That's how fast it happened; the decision seemed to make itself. I only knew about heroin from what I'd seen in movies and read in books. I knew it got you to the kind of high that erased the world around you, and I wanted that, needed that, and that need superseded any rationale, any potential consequence. I wanted an exit door. And I thought heroin might be it.

Yes, I want to get high; I want to feel anything else other than ev-erything I have ever felt.

From my seat on the floor, resting against the bed, I watched Ted as he sat at his desk and cooked the heroin in a spoon. It smelled sweet but nauseating, like coffee and shoe polish and sugar, all gone a little rotten. My heart was beating so fast as I offered him my arm. He had to give me my shot first before taking one himself. He wrapped a belt around my arm and told me to pump my fist as he felt the crook of my arm for the right spot, dabbing it with a small alcohol wipe. *I love the way his hands feel.* The needle went in with the slightest sting and the moment happened—the moment the heroin hit my bloodstream for the first time. I tasted rubbing alcohol and a cloying sweetness in the back of my throat.

Then the world dropped out from beneath me.

Everything sped up, zoomed through me, played back in slow motion. I saw him back at his desk, then closed my eyes, opened them, and felt his breath on my cheek, losing myself in the deep green pools of his eyes. I was walking underwater; I felt everything and nothing. I closed my eyes again. I opened my eyes, and he was floating through me. I let him take me, take my virginity in a flurry that blinded me, like staring at the sun. There were no concrete sensations. It was all abstract, all outside me. The one thought that pulsed in the back of my mind was, *Somehow this is familiar, somehow you were never a virgin.*

Siouxsie sang, "But oh, your city lies in dust, my friend," and she joined me underwater. I felt my life vacuumed up at that moment, sealed and put on a shelf somewhere far away where I couldn't see it, and I liked it. Disconnected from my body, disconnected from the room around me, I drifted. I drifted away from Ted, from the walls and the floor of his room. I felt I could spend an eternity like that, just drifting, where nobody could touch me because I remained in motion.

Then, suddenly, I had motion sickness. I dropped out of the air and back into my body, and I knew I was going to be sick. I fell out of the bed and rushed, stumbling naked, to the bathroom, making it just in time. I puked. I puked and I puked and I puked until there was nothing left of me. I lay on the cold marble floor and reminded myself to breathe. After what might have been two minutes or two hours, I got up, brushed my teeth with my finger, and put my mouth to the faucet, gulping down water, then went back to bed.

Ted was nodded out. I climbed in next to him and let myself drift again, marveling at this distance I felt from myself. And just like that, heroin entered my life.

CHAPTER 2
Swimming Horses
July 1987

Poseidon, god of the sea, was also the king of horses. They led him over the surface of the ocean. Swimming horses, not seahorses. You can find them at the Trevi Fountain in Rome. You can make a wish there, and maybe they will carry you somewhere, across the surface of an ocean.

Every July, since 1925, wild horses swim from one island to the next across the Assateague Channel when the tide is "slack calm." From Chincoteague to Assateague and back again, they swim. But I was nowhere near the Assateague Channel.

I spent my thirteenth summer working for Albert, a well-known horse trainer. I spent all day, every day, from 7:00 a.m. until the sun went down, riding the horses of people who were too busy to ride them. The only time I remember being happy that summer was there, riding those horses, sharing my secrets with them.

I stared at the bright blue blinking numbers on my white cube alarm clock. It was 6:29. One more minute. Unsure of how long

I had been staring at the numbers, my mind was stuck in a circle. The radio alarm still managed to startle me, playing Echo & The Bunnymen's "Bring on the Dancing Horses."

Knowing I had ten—no, nine—minutes to get out the door, I grabbed my jeans and tank top and tiptoed down the hall, stopping to peek into my mother's bedroom. Relief. The Asshole had already left for work. He and my mom had made it through their rough patch; my hatred for him had only grown over the past six months.

Whenever he spoke to me, I could feel—really, I could hear—the disdain in his voice. Last December, the three of us had gone to see *The Nutcracker* and he was angry about traffic, muttering under his breath. When he was agitated like that, my mom became still and silent. I wanted to do the same but I couldn't; I felt a compulsion to fill the hostile silence with words, so I yammered on with any kind of small talk I could think of. At a stoplight, he turned around and snapped at me, "Erin, can you stop talking? Just shut up."

My mom said nothing, and I felt heat rise to the surface of my skin. It burned and I didn't know who I hated more in that moment, him or her. My grandfather had been like this with my mom, but worse. I knew that, or knew some of it, and I tried to let that excuse her for remaining frozen in those moments, the ones when his anger lashed out at me against all the parts of me I wished my mom could see.

Then there was the time earlier that spring when he was helping me with my algebra homework. When I didn't understand what he was trying to explain, he threw everything off the breakfast table and stormed away. I sat there watching the pieces of paper slowly float to the floor—unable to process what I had done wrong, but knowing I had come up short in some way.

Mornings like this when he was already gone for the day were a reprieve. The air felt different, like it could actually circulate. I heard my mom downstairs in the kitchen. She'd packed my lunch in a little blue-and-white cooler. I loved that little cooler; it reminded me that I was leaving. Every morning, I felt excited about the prospect of what might be in there, but I only ate the apricots. Sometimes, I fed the leftovers to Lisette, a Lipizzan mare I'd been assigned to ride. I hated riding her. She was still a little wild and continually tried to buck me off. We had an antagonistic relationship but I understood her. She made sense. She wasn't a labyrinth disguised as a straight line.

I waited in the dining room for my mom. The dining room was the only room in the house that felt safe—maybe it was because it was close to the front door, close to an exit, maybe it was because I used to talk to my imaginary friend there, or maybe it was because it housed my favorite painting. Sometimes, when I couldn't sleep, I'd go down there and lie on the table and look at that painting. The sky in the painting was inky blue and the house with the red door looked like somewhere I would like to be. I wanted to tuck away, small and secure, far away from people who were labyrinths disguised as straight lines. I was the worst offender. I wanted to get away from me, too, more than I was with my weekend escapes into the warm arms of heroin. And Ted. I shut my eyes and imagined that house on Chincoteague, imagined that I could see the swimming horses from that window.

On the drive to the barn, Mom and I made small talk.

"So how are things going with Albert?" she asked.

"Fine. Good."

"This summer is such a great experience for you, honey. I'm so glad you decided to do this."

"Yeah. I'm really learning a lot."

Our morning conversations were usually like this. She'd comment on my summer or the weather or her workouts, or if I was going to make weekend plans with my father when he was in from New York, or what to eat for dinner, or what she put in that little blue-and-white cooler for my lunch. Whatever she said, I'd agree and comment back politely.

What I didn't tell her was it was the most confusing summer of my life. I didn't tell her that I was hiding more and more parts of myself. I was hiding a boyfriend and drugs and cuts on my arms and secrets I carried from a long time ago. I didn't tell her that every day I woke up and went to the barn and lost myself in the scent of horse sweat and alfalfa and leather and dirt and wood. And those horses and grounding smells made me feel like maybe I wouldn't disappear. Instead, I kissed her goodbye and got out of the car.

The barn seemed too quiet. Albert was large and cranky and walked with a cane. It was hard to imagine that he ever rode a horse. His wife, Mimi, reminded me of those photos of young Priscilla Presley, with the big hair and the eyeliner and the swingy clothes. She was stuck in some other time, maybe some other place, too, and was younger than Albert's only daughter, Jolene.

Jolene was red in the face with disappointment. She had white-blond hair and eyes that betrayed the injuries she carried, though I never found out exactly what those were. I was thirteen and Jolene was thirty-three, but we connected because we were broken.

The door to Albert's office swung open with determination and Jolene stormed toward me. Albert's voice followed, loud and fast, like a hot angry wind behind her. She brushed past me. Her face was purple, and I looked at the ground, silent. Mimi came out next like an apologetic puff of air and diverted me to the tack room, chatting about the schedule and how June gloom had bled into July.

"MIMI!" Albert shouted from down the breezeway.

Mimi scurried back to the office and I headed to Dom's stall. Dom was a large black Hanoverian warmblood. He was the most beautiful horse in the barn and I got to ride him every day because his owner was afraid to ride him. I cleaned out his hooves with a hoof pick and used a currycomb on his coat. Then I leaned on him; I let all my weight rest on his shoulder, breathing in. I thought about the lie I was going to come up with to cover my tracks the next weekend when I went to Ted's.

For the past eight or nine months, I'd been cleverly coming up with stories about where I went and who I was staying with. Sometimes I told my mom I was staying with Lisa, my closest friend from school. Sometimes I told her I was staying with Rhea, a friend from the barn. Sometimes I'd be where I said I was going to be. But she never checked, and as the months rolled on, I was in Ted's bed more and more, floating on a cloud of nothing.

I didn't take drugs home with me. I hadn't gotten that bold. In between cheerleading and volleyball and horseback riding and school, I counted the days and minutes until I was back in that all-white house, looking down at twinkling lights below, drifting. His parents were rarely home and when they were, they treated me like a friendly ghost, never quite looking at me or Ted when they spoke. Maybe they were the ghosts.

Sometimes, during the week, I'd steal another Darvocet from the expired bottle in our medicine cabinet. Sometimes I'd look through other people's medicine cabinets and I'd take a pill or two if I found anything good. And when I couldn't do that, I took a small razor blade and made tiny marks on the inside of my arm, cutting, mesmerized by the appearance of microscopic trails of blood coming to the surface to greet me. It wasn't heroin, but it softened the hardened shape I found myself in, trapped in all of the perfunctory crap I smiled my way through every day. My life was becoming a series of compartments connected by a long string of lies and duplicities, of pretending to be all the versions of me they wanted, or I thought they wanted.

I felt like everyone in my life needed a different Erin. My parents needed the daughter who didn't need anything, the one who wasn't difficult or sad, the one who brought home good grades and was polite and pretty and made them look like they were doing everything right. My trainers needed me to ride and win riding competitions and take their corrections and show up every day. My friends needed me to make them laugh and give them advice and not be a drag. Ted needed me to make him feel wanted and to make him feel loved and not ask too many questions. And me, I needed me to keep pushing and acting and shining and sparkling in every area of my life. If I did that, if I was all those things, then no one would see what was crumbling and rotten on the inside.

Here I am pretending to take a test. Oh, look, I got an A! Here I am laughing at Eddie's joke during lunch. Here I am at volleyball practice. Here I am at Lisa's house, gossiping, obsessing over boys, and not mentioning Ted. Here I am in the ring, riding a stubborn mare. Here I am in the barn, inhaling the smells that keep me from leaving. Here I am at a sleepover at Rhea's, devising a way to leave early to go to Ted's. And here I am fantasizing, plotting slow and painful ways to kill my mother's arrogant, asshole boyfriend—a favorite pastime when I couldn't sleep, which was often.

The one person who anchored me to who I was before the drugs was my grandma—my mom's mom. Since my parents had separated years before, I'd regularly gone to Grandma's apartment after school to do my homework, eat dinner, and wait for my mom to pick me up. Grandma was everything my mom was not. She was fat and had bold red hair that she had done at the "beauty parlor." I felt that my mom was embarrassed by her, of the ways she did or didn't take care of herself. But to me she was magic. She was love. I didn't understand then their own complicated mother–daughter relationship.

While my mom spent her evenings at the gym, perfecting her already thin body, Grandma and I watched *Dynasty* and *T.J. Hooker* and music videos on MTV. She smoked long, thin brown cigarettes and made me pepper steak, and macaroni and

cheese, and fruit salad with Cool Whip and marshmallows—
food that would never be served at home because at home we
only ate "healthy" food.

I loved her. I loved her smile and her blue eyeshadow and her
fluffy white couch and her small dark apartment and the way
she smelled—Jean Naté drugstore after-bath body splash and
cigarettes and cheap lipstick and face powder. Grandma was the
strongest sense of home I had. But even she didn't know about
the drugs. She did know about Ted, sort of. I'd mentioned him
to her, downplaying the time I spent with him. I made her swear
not to tell my mom. And she didn't. As I spent more time at
the barn and lying to see Ted, I spent less time with her. I was
pulling away from my anchor and it was painful, but I couldn't
stop myself.

Jolene was in the stall next door. I smelled her clove cigarette, and I asked her, over the wall, about the schedule. I didn't
tell her that Mimi already told me. I talked too much because
I knew she was sad. I wanted to fill the silences to distract us
both, so I asked her if she'd ever seen the swimming horses.
She'd never heard of them.

"We should go together to see them," I told her. "Maybe we
haven't missed it yet. It's this month!"

"Well, if I took a vacation that would be right up my alley.
But I don't take vacations, sweets. Never. Ever."

I walked around to the stall she was in and looked at her. Her
hair was so light; it stuck to her face like a sweaty halo. She finally looked up. I wanted to hug her, tell her I understood her
hurt, tell her she was like a big sister to me. In my thirteen-
year-old logic, I thought if I could help her, that meant there
was hope for me, too. Instead, I smiled and told her I was taking Dom out.

Dom and I went on a trail ride and as I sang to him, my voice
carried more than melody. It carried the wounds and the pain-

ful silences I held. He listened and we understood each other. I clucked my tongue and urged him forward into a canter.

The wind whipping through my hair and licking my face, I ride. I ride with a certainty I don't possess in life. My heart knows the way, I shut my eyes. I share my secrets. I see swimming horses. They carry me across the surface of an ocean.

CHAPTER 3
Eucalyptus
November 1987

I was cramped, curled up next to Kasey in the back of my mom's Saab, waiting for her. Kasey was our huge white German shepherd, who was untrustworthy and bit people. Even still, he made me feel safe locked in that car on a dark street in Silverlake on a late Sunday night. My mom was inside The Asshole's house, talking. He had days before broken up with my mom because "he couldn't be with someone who had the baggage she had." Meaning, the kind of baggage that was almost fourteen and talked too much and wasn't great at algebra and looked just like her father.

My mom did not handle this breakup well. She spiraled into the place she'd been in after her father died, the place that scared me when I was four. She stopped eating, she cried all the time, she begged me not to go to school because she didn't want to be alone. And on this particular Sunday night, she drove over to The Asshole's house to talk. To beg? To try to win someone back who didn't deserve her to begin with. And it made me sick. And it made me sad. Why she insisted on bringing me, I don't know. But there I was, in the back of her Saab, with my very own bodyguard—Kasey.

Thankfully, *Loveline* was on. *Loveline* was a call-in radio show that aired late at night on KROQ, an alternative radio station in LA. Everyone I knew listened to Dr. Drew and "The Poorman" dispensing advice to their callers. I usually tuned in from the comfort of my bed, but tonight it was in the Saab. It's funny to think about how years later Dr. Drew would be my doctor in rehab and that even more years later, I would be the one doling out advice on life like they did.

That night, a young woman phoned in, afraid she was pregnant. She was sixteen. As they talked her through family planning options, it dawned on me that I'd been sleeping with Ted for almost a year. We almost never used a condom. *We have to start using condoms. Or maybe the pill. Something. Maybe I can't get pregnant*, I thought, which was rationalized from nothing but the overwhelming feeling that I would be a horrible mother. I didn't want kids. I'd felt sure of this since I'd been a little girl playing with my Cabbage Patch doll. I loved her, but even then, I felt disconnected from any maternal longing that most little girls, like all my friends, experienced.

The minutes ticked on into hours while I waited for my mom. When a car would come down the street—or worse, a person walking by—I'd lie as flat as I could, hugging Kasey, scared of what might be lurking in the dark outside. What I was really scared of was who would come back to the car after this "talk" my mom was having. Would she come back more broken than before? Or would they get back together, The Asshole moving back in with us?

My mom flung the driver's side door open, crying, and started the car. I didn't say a word. I was immobile—frozen and flat, clutching Kasey. She sobbed all the way home, struggling not to hyperventilate.

The weeks that followed were brutal. My mom was inconsolable. I often stayed home from school, fearful that she might take her own life if I left her alone for very long. I'd also come to suspect that she blamed me. Sometimes she'd make an off-hand remark about me not being nice to The Asshole when he lived with us. Every time she did this, it was like she was choosing him instead of me.

I wanted to scream in her face, rattle off the long list of times he'd yelled at me, belittled me, "put me in my place." I wanted to ask, "What about me? Don't you love me more?" Instead, I continued to withdraw, all the while acting like everything was normal—just fine, just as it should be. I had to. Underneath the anger I had toward my mom for not protecting me was the fear that it *was* my fault—that my ugliness, my brokenness, ruined everything around me, even my mother's relationship. The larger that fear swelled inside me, the more frantic I became to find a way to pretend everything was okay.

Around the holidays, I felt my depression suck me into that deep well, right alongside her. And I hated her for it. When school let out the week before Christmas, I crossed the first of many imaginary lines I'd set for myself—I brought heroin home. It was powdered, which meant I could snort it. I didn't bring a needle home. Powdered heroin was rare in LA, but Ted's brother had procured it from wherever it was he went for college, somewhere on the East Coast. Ted and I took some from his stash and he insisted I take some with me. He knew things at home were rough. I'd use at night, after my mom had gone to bed, and let myself drift, let myself escape for a while. That release was the only thing I looked forward to.

On Christmas Eve, my dad came over to pick me up and take us to the annual Christmas Eve party of our good family friends Ken and Olga. He also came to check on my mom. When my parents split up, the absence of my father hadn't been a huge change, as he had already been traveling for work back and forth between New York and California for some time. And now he had a condo at the beach, so he was technically back in California every weekend, though I didn't see him that often.

One thing my parents were not good at was a clean break. I wasn't sure why my parents had separated, but their separation and their lack of boundaries afterward was a pattern I would replicate with my own relationships. And much as when they'd been married, when my mom was in crisis, my dad liked to step in, be the hero.

My mom didn't want to go to the party, but I was afraid to leave her. She was upstairs in her office, on the phone with The Asshole. I could hear the muffled sounds of arguing and more tears. I was sick of the tears. So, so sick of them. My dad and I sat downstairs, the silence heavy between us. We had been awkward around each other for the past couple of years, but the backdrop of my mom's drama amplified the awkwardness.

I looked up at him. My dad was objectively handsome. I used to tease him that he was an older, shorter, slightly less attractive version of George Clooney. Women always loved my dad and found him charming. He was charming. He was the guy who commanded a room when he walked in, in a totally friendly and approachable way. Yet, as his daughter, he didn't feel approachable. We looked so much alike that I wondered if when he looked at me he saw all the things he didn't like about himself. I wondered if he'd wished I looked like my mom: golden and angular and light. He was whistling, looking away, thinking about something else. I opened my mouth to start a conversation when I heard my mom throw something. And then another something.

I shot up the stairs, my anger fueled by the days and weeks of tears and offhand remarks of blame. My dad followed behind. My mom stood in her office, in the center of her own storm. I marched up to her, I grabbed her by the shoulders, and screamed in her face, "Snap out of it!" and slapped her.

Every molecule of oxygen suspended in the air around us. No one moved. No one said anything. The air was so still. In the end, she promised she would be there when we returned and my dad and I did go to the party. He told me, years later, that he was shocked; he realized at that moment how bad things had been, which is probably why he ended up sticking close to us in the days that followed.

Christmas Day was spent at my mom's best friend's house. My dad came. Grandma was there, too. Grandma was famous (or infamous, if you asked my mom) for her bright and glittered wrapping. She used to write my name in big looping glue letters and then pour silver or gold or red or green glitter on top of them. Months after the wrapping paper and Christmas tree had been thrown away, little pieces of glitter remained, discreet, appearing suddenly in a corner of the Persian rug. It irritated my mom to no end. This year there was no glitter, and when I opened her card to me, I teased her because she addressed the card to herself and signed it "Love, Erin." She seemed a little off. This wasn't like her. As we ate dinner, I pushed my food around, preoccupied with how much dope I had back home that I'd saved for myself as a Christmas present.

The following day, my dad took me and my mom to Lake Tahoe for a last-minute getaway. My friend Rhea came with us. Because it was last-minute, and this was in the dark ages before Airbnb or Expedia or easy access to the internet, we ended up in a condo for the night that no one seemed happy about. The condo was all dark wood and pea green curtains and felt like no one had been there for quite some time. It had a musty smell, and with the heat on, it felt stifling.

It was late; we were all tired from the long day of driving, and I had trouble sleeping. Even though I wasn't fully strung out—I was still controlling and dabbling—the past few days of snorting heroin every night before bed had disrupted my circadian rhythm. As the hours rolled slowly along, I drifted in and out of sleep—hot, restless, and having difficulty breathing.

Around 4:00 a.m., I jumped up, hysterical, gasping for air, waking everyone up.

"Go back to sleep!" my mother snapped at me.

Everyone was angry. But I couldn't breathe. I felt like I was dying.

"I can't breathe. I can't breathe." I repeated this, my thoughts in a circle that got tighter and tighter.

I was shaking and panting and my limbs went numb. A buzzing pressure pushed down all around my head and heat swelled up to the surface of my skin.

"You're fine. Just go back to bed," I think someone said.

I did what I'd been doing since I was a very young child. I went to the bathroom, locked the door, and lay on the floor, letting the cool tile hold the weight of me. After some time, my breathing slowed down, and as the feeling came back into my limbs, the tingling was replaced by profound sadness. I thought I was crazy. I couldn't tell them what I was feeling. I didn't have words for it. I got back into bed and stayed as still as possible and held my breath and counted.

The next afternoon, we checked into Harrah's Hotel and Casino in South Lake Tahoe. It was a relief to leave the condo for a huge suite, the excitement of a casino beneath us—something my dad loved. I remember being so amused by the telephones in the bathrooms. We joked about yapping away on the phone while pooping.

We hadn't been in the room for long when the phone rang. My mom kidded about the fact that she was answering it from the bathroom. It was my cousin Kristin. She was dog-sitting Kasey for us. I heard my mother shriek, or I think I heard her shriek; maybe I just sensed it. I opened the bathroom door. My mom dropped the phone. There was a flurry of movement and voices and the room swirled around me and somewhere in all of it, I heard it.

"My mother is dead. My mother is dead."

It took me a minute to make that critical connection. *Grandma.* MY beloved grandma, my home, my heart, was dead. The sound of Mom's voice—"my mother is dead"—resounded in my ears. And I felt angry, so angry at my mother, who had never treated Grandma well enough, never appreciated her enough, had never loved her the way I did. *How dare she be crying.* And then I felt angry at myself—for being distant, for spending Christmas thinking about heroin in my last moments with her.

We checked out and made the long drive back to Los Angeles, in a snowstorm. It was silent inside that car. Rhea held my hand and I grabbed on and didn't let go.

In the days before the funeral, I felt nothing—not anger or sadness, just an aching emptiness. I went to Rhea's, I went to Lisa's, and I went to Ted's. I brought home more dope to snort at night before bed; Ted was always generous. I'd been so reluctant, for almost a year, to bring heroin home with me; it would make it too real. But once I crossed that line, I didn't hesitate.

I avoided most interaction with my mother, which wasn't hard to do with my dad and family friends keeping her occupied. It was unclear how Grandma died. She had health problems for years: diabetes and high blood pressure and heart disease. The official cause of death was cardiac arrest or natural causes. My uncle, my mom's brother, who'd handled things, didn't order an autopsy. We did learn that she'd died exactly at the time I'd woken up screaming, unable to breathe. I am certain that I felt it when she died. She took a part of me with her. I feared she took the only good part left.

The day of Grandma's funeral arrived. My mom was shaky, my dad by her side, and I was still feeling empty as we stood outside the little chapel high atop a hill above Forest Lawn. The Asshole showed up, looking repentant, wearing his stupid cowboy boots. He wasn't a fucking cowboy. My emptiness turned to hate. During the service, I held it together sitting in the front pew. The leftover high from days of snorting heroin flattening me just enough.

At the end of the service, we filed past Grandma's open casket. The second I saw her bright red hair, teased and sprayed in a bouffant, sticking out of the top of the coffin, I collapsed. Sara, the daughter of our good family friends Ken and Olga, ran up and collected me, walking me out as I leaned with all my weight on her small frame. Outside the chapel, I started bawling, finally letting out all the devastation I'd been suppressing. Instead of coming to comfort me, I watched as Mom walked over to talk to The Asshole.

Sara sat with me on the curb, her arm around me, hugging me. I glared at my mom. After a short conversation, my mom hugged him goodbye and The Asshole left. But I wondered what this meant. Would he be back again?

Later at home, after everyone had left and it was just the two of us, I knocked on my mom's door.

"Mom?"

"Yeah?" She sounded so small.

I got up on her bed and lay down next to her, put my head on her chest. She petted my hair and I exhaled with relief. It was the first time in weeks, maybe months, that I felt like some semblance of the mom I needed still existed.

"Are you doing okay?" she asked.

"Yeah, I'm okay. Can I ask you something? Are you getting back together with him?"

She stopped petting my hair, sat up a bit, and said, "No. No, honey, I'm not."

I wasn't sure if I could believe her.

While my mom and I weren't as close as before, things stabilized at home. She remained true to her word—The Asshole was gone from our lives. My dad bought me a new horse. Ranson was a gorgeous dappled gray Trakehner warmblood gelding—

a jumper, trained by an Olympic coach. I switched trainers and barns, choosing a quieter, smaller barn where my new friend Ellen kept her horse. Mom forged new friendships with my trainers, easing the pressure off of me to fill her time, to be her friend. My love of riding and horses continued to help contain my drug use, another compartment to keep things under control. By spring, I spent as much time as possible out of the house—at the barn, at school, at Ted's, at Rhea's, and increasingly with Sam, Ted's cousin.

Sam was with Ted when we met. We were the same age, and he also dabbled with drugs but not as much as Ted and I did. He was Ted-lite. Ted without the edges. Ted without the suspicion that I was being lied to. Ted cheated on me with increasing frequency. I didn't love him, but I'd wanted him to love me. Survival skills, old ones, emerged—*if I keep a straight face, if I keep moving, if I never stop, no one can hurt me.* I took any hurt I felt and turned it inward, spitting it back out as apathy. And the drugs he was dispensing did a good job of letting me slide right underneath any feelings I might have had.

As Sam and I spent more and more time together, he became my new confidant, my safe place. In that teenage way, we became quickly glued to one another, and I kept murky boundaries with him that weren't fair to either one of us. We flirted and tempted each other to cross that line of friendship to something more. Increasingly, it was Sam I thought about—his mop of light brown hair, his saucerlike hazel eyes that looked at me with a kindness I wasn't used to. We spent countless nights talking on the phone about Morrissey, and The Jesus and Mary Chain, and how we were obsessed with *Beetlejuice.* We talked about meeting up at KROQ's daytime Mighty Lemon Drops concert, about going to Magic Mountain over spring break, and if I should get bangs. Sometimes, we talked about how I should break up with Ted, stop doing drugs. He told me I deserved better. And sometimes I believed him.

One night in May, I hung out with Sam in Toluca Lake after riding. We took a couple of Vicodin I'd stolen and went for a walk on the quiet streets of his neighborhood. We passed by the house of my new friend from the barn, Ellen. We stopped outside her house and I debated knocking, but we kept walking. I wanted to be alone with him. The streets felt deserted. I don't think we saw a single person, a single car—or we didn't notice them—as we laughed and talked and held hands.

We passed by Bob Hope's estate and found a quiet spot of sidewalk flanked by eucalyptus trees. We lay in the grass and Sam kissed me. I kissed him back and then pulled away.

"We have one skinny old eucalyptus tree in front of my house," I said, "and when the Santa Anas kick up, it sways so violently, I swear one day it's going to snap in two. I kind of hate it."

He brushed the hair away from my eyes and kissed me again. Again, I kissed him back and pulled away.

"You know, eucalyptus trees aren't even supposed to be in California. Australian dudes brought them here during the Gold Rush," I blabbered on.

I made a dumb joke about koala bears that I can't remember. I did what I would do over and over in years to come: I let someone in, while also pushing them away—not letting them go. It's a dangerous way to play with someone's heart, and yet, I couldn't stop myself. And Sam, *oh, Sam*, he was only too willing to let me.

July 4, 1988

I spent the Fourth of July with Lisa at her friend's house in Orange County. She, like me, was in the habit of using plans with friends as a ruse for seeing her older boyfriend. Yet I still concealed my relationship with Ted from her, and had been for a year and a half. Her boyfriend never showed and we got drunk on White Russians. Funny enough, it was the first time I'd been drunk, ever. I hated it. It felt hard and clumsy; heroin always felt soft.

Ted and I weren't speaking. I knew he was cheating on me again. But I was more upset by my fight with Sam that morning. I'd called him because I needed to vent. Ted had stood me up, disappeared, and I was hurt. I knew I didn't love Ted, and maybe it was all ego, but it stung, and I felt that familiar rejection that lodged in my gut. That feeling for me, that feeling of rejection, has always taken space right up against my diaphragm, like a vise closing in slowly and steadily. Sam barely had a chance to say hello before I launched into a tirade.

"Ted says he was with you last night. Is this true?" I asked.

"What?" he replied, buying time to come up with an answer.

"Sam, was he with you last night?"

"Yes."

"Are you lying to me?"

"If you are so sure he's lying, why do you fucking stay?"

"I know you're lying to me," I said through hot, angry tears.

"I really don't know what to say. You're fucking lying to him, too. Or do you think he'd be cool with you and me fooling around all the time?"

"We haven't slept together!" I snapped, indignant.

"Oh, I know—I'm the one who stupidly keeps coming back to be tortured and used."

"You think I'm using you?" I asked.

"Aren't you?"

I was livid. He was right. After that first kiss on the grass in Toluca Lake, we'd been playing out a dance of advancement and retreat. We kissed, we fondled, I pulled back. I left him frustrated and confused. The fact that I was fooling around with him and still stayed with Ted in a decidedly unhealthy relationship became too much—for Sam, and for me.

He continued, "Let's see, you call me whenever you're mad

at Ted. I listen. I bite my tongue. My cousin is a piece of shit. You know this, yet you stay. You know I'm fucking in love with you, and what do you do? You play with my head. I am done doing this. You want to stay with some asshole that treats you like shit, that doesn't even know the real you? Be my guest. But I am not gonna be your consolation prize when Ted fucks you over again and again."

My skin was on fire, I felt like I was choking on his words—the truth—and I said, "Yeah? Well, fuck you then," and hung up the phone.

On July 5, Lisa and I gathered our things from her friend's house and rode home, hungover, with her mom, who'd come to pick us up. I was dehydrated, my head throbbed, and I was still obsessing over that phone call with Sam. When I got home, I hurried to my bedroom, sure that Sam left me a message; I was fortunate to have a private phone line. Sure enough, the light on my answering machine was blinking away. Six messages. The first was from Lisa when I was en route to her house. The second was a hang-up. The third was Sam, speaking slurred, loud music in the background—The Cure's "Close to Me." I couldn't make out what he said. The fourth was another hang-up. The fifth was Ted; he sounded strange, like his voice was trapped inside another answering machine and being played back. The sixth message was Ted again. His voice cracked. "Call me. As soon as you get this. Something's happened. Call me."

I knew. I knew somewhere deep in my body that it was about Sam. That the "something's happened" was about Sam. I wish I could say I'd been wrong. I wish I could go back in time and rewrite the events. But I couldn't. I can't.

Sam was dead. He'd had a brain aneurysm while I was watching fireworks from a backyard in Orange County, drunk on White Russians. As Ted spoke on the phone, my ears rang and I felt all the air around me evaporate. Everything compressed. Everything sucked dry.

"Can I come over?" I asked.

"Where do you want me to pick you up?"

I told my mom I was going riding and then to Rhea's. She dropped me at the barn and Ted picked me up there. We went back to his parentless white house and got high and had sex for the first time in a month. I wanted the drugs, I wanted his body, I wanted anything and everything to lay on me, move through me, press all the secrets and lies and loss and grief of the past several months away. I'd lost Grandma a little over six months ago. And now Sam. That loss scratched around inside me, the way it had after Grandma died.

The next morning, Ted dropped me off back at the barn. I met up with Rhea for a trail ride. When she had to head back to the barn, I kept riding. I rode through Griffith Park, on my usual trails, past the creeps. On almost every trail ride, some pervert would appear; I'd come to expect it. I'd been taught to ignore them. I rode past the naked jogger, the flasher, the masturbator hiding in the shrubs. I didn't care. I looked at them all, daring them to come at me. That's the thing about grief—sometimes it's so sharp, you feel fearless. I wondered how far Ranson and I could go. I wondered if he could carry me across the surface of an ocean.

CHAPTER 4
Somedays
Summer 1988

The grief I felt after losing Grandma returned with Sam's death. At moments, I couldn't separate the two losses and felt large, hollow spaces open inside me. Their deaths haunted me and somehow the drugs weren't enough to provide me relief. I had to try to push forward in another way.

Ellen and I grew closer, spending long days at the barn together. Much like it had been with Sam, my attachment to Ellen was quick and all-consuming. We were opposites in many ways. She was petite and fair and an open book; I was tall and dark and held in so many parts of me. I was enamored with her in that teenage girl-crush sort of way. And our friendship, while maybe all encompassing, was exactly what I needed—it let me be fourteen.

I was focused on my riding. I spent hours grooming horses, listening to Morrissey's *Viva Hate* on repeat on my little Sony boom box, mourning the loss of Sam as I inhaled the comforting smell of sweat and dirt and hay and leather. All I wanted was to disconnect from the secrecy and pain of the months before.

Yet, I didn't share my grief with anyone, at least not in any real way. I mentioned it to Ellen—that I'd lost a friend. But I didn't tell her how or why or what he meant to me.

I didn't want to go back to my old prep school in the fall. Outside Lisa, I didn't care about any of my friends there, and she was transferring to another school. A new school felt like a clean break, a fresh start; I could leave the heroin and secrets and lies behind me. My mom listened and enrolled me into a new school, close to the barn, where Ellen went. With The Asshole out of the picture, my mom was present in ways like this—taking care of business and paying attention to my needs. Even though I was processing the sorrow of all the losses, I felt hopeful.

By mid-August, weeks had passed without me touching drugs. And weeks without touching Ted. We'd barely seen each other. After Sam died, he'd gone on vacation to Hawaii with his family. Now he was back and his grief spun off him like shrapnel. He was *not* done with drugs. As my drug use came to a halt, his accelerated and included freebasing cocaine and acting more and more erratic. Our phone calls became him yelling at my pillow, where I'd dropped the phone.

On a swampy August night, out of excuses, I'd agreed to see him, knowing that I needed to end things. He picked me up at our usual dark corner, around the bend from the barn. He was high. He was flying. He'd lost weight and the angles of his face were too sharp. He was tan from Hawaii but somehow still looked ashen. I didn't want to get stuck all the way in Beverly Hills with him driving. Instead, I convinced him to go down the road to Viva Rancho Cantina, a kitschy Mexican restaurant next to the LA Equestrian Center. The thought crossed my mind that I might run into my horse trainers or someone else from the barn, but being able to walk away from him and not be trapped in Beverly Hills was worth the risk.

As soon as we were seated, a waiter slapped a basket of chips and some salsa down, along with the menus and two glasses of water in dark red plastic cups. Ted put his hand under the table and squeezed my thigh, rubbing it up and down, as I watched a trail of water trickle down the table and off the edge. I tensed when he touched me, and he felt it.

"What's up with you?" he asked.

"I don't know. I just feel weird about things," I said.

He jumped up and said, "I'll be right back."

Ted went to the bathroom and came back with a wild yet vacant look in his eyes. It's that coked-out look, when someone is all lit up, but they're not there. They look past you, can't see you. *Would he even be able to process that I'm breaking up with him?*

We placed our order, but I knew I wasn't waiting until the end of this meal.

"I think I need a break," I said.

He stared past me.

"From us."

He looked at me now. "What does that mean?"

"I just need some space. And you do, too. I know you're sleeping around."

He opened his mouth, looking ready to defend himself, but looked down instead and dropped his chip.

"Well, then, what the fuck are we doing here..." he said to the table.

I pushed my chair back, and it made a loud noise, loud enough to cause people to look, which was impressive for such a noisy restaurant. I stood up. Ted kept staring at the table. I went to touch his shoulder on the way out, then pulled back, and said, "I'm sorry."

Walking out of Viva, I felt like I could breathe again, like I'd only been taking shallow breaths for as long as I could remember. I walked back to the stables. Ellen was still there, and I asked if I could spend the night. We went back to her house. I loved her parents. Her dad was a cameraman and looked like a movie star. Her mom was an adorable middle-aged Brigitte

Bardot type, a former actress herself. They always made me feel welcome in their home.

Ellen's dad took us to rent movies and get frozen yogurt from a place we loved in a strip mall on Moorpark. Like always, I got peach-banana. We stayed up late, watching *The Witches of East-wick* and laughing a lot. For the first time since I started using drugs, I felt normal.

As the remainder of summer ticked forward, my world revolved around horses, and Ellen and I became inseparable. I spent all my time at her house or the barn and was genuinely excited for the new school year, a fresh start with my new best friend. But something else was happening—I was starting to feel things again.

The thick protective coating that heroin had provided was gone. And I was left with all the difficult feelings I had avoided—grief over the loss of Grandma and Sam, unresolved anger toward my parents, and scariest of all, that nagging unnamed fear that lived in the pit of my stomach. It came from foggy memories and summoned a strong sense of shame from all the sexual parts of my body.

My first day at my new school started like many—rushed. Getting out the door, my mom was moving too slowly and I was irritated. We sat in traffic on the exit ramp from the 134 Freeway and she seemed unfazed, sipping her coffee. I let out a loud sigh, arguably one of my more annoying passive-aggressive moves, one I still struggle to let go of today.

"What's that for?" she asked.

"What?"

"The sigh."

I rolled my eyes and looked out the window. "Nothing. I didn't..."

"What time should I pick you up today?"

"You're not."

"I'm not?"

"No, I'm going to the barn with Ellen and then I'm going to spend the night at her house."

"On a school night?"

"I asked you about this, Mom. Jesus."

"Erin, watch your tone."

"I don't have a tone, Mother. I asked you. You said yes. It's not my fault you don't remember."

As we pulled in the driveway of my new school, I could see my mom's lips tighten out of the corner of my eye as she gripped the wheel.

"Well, I just thought it would be nice to hear about your first day and have dinner together tonight," she said.

"God, I miss the days when all you cared about was your stupid boyfriend."

I got out of the car and swung the door shut before she could answer.

It was becoming more and more difficult to talk with my mom, much less have a close relationship. I lashed out at her frequently; I seemed irrational. I made jabs at her about her ex-boyfriend. I didn't want to see my dad. I felt impatient and angry with him for his absence, for his inability to protect me from my mom, and for showing up for her in ways I thought he never would for me.

Without the drugs, my mood swings became intense and did not go unnoticed. My mom found a therapist for me, Dr. Geoffrey. He reminded me of this actor on that show *China Beach*, which my mom and I started watching earlier that year. I liked his blue blazers and brown leather loafers and the Chesterfield sofa in his office. I liked his ordinariness, his kind eyes, and I adored him because he listened to me. More important, he heard me. I told Dr. Geoffrey about Ted. I told him about the drugs I'd done. I told him about struggling with suicidal feelings. And I told him about that nagging feeling in my stomach, and how it made me feel ashamed all the time.

On a mild Saturday evening in early October, I was back home from the barn, sticky with the residue of a day on and around horses. My trainers had dropped me off; my mom was out of town for the weekend. I sat down on the edge of my bed and pressed Play on my little white answering machine, its angry red light blinking. There were several messages from Ted. He was crying, he was pleading, then he was angry, then subdued and sounding high. As I sat there trying to process what it all meant, my phone rang. I shouldn't have picked it up, but I did.

"I need to see you," Ted said before I even got the word *hello* out of my mouth.

"I feel like that's not a good idea."

"Please, please, I'm having a really hard time."

"I'm sorry," I said.

"The coroner's report came back. They found drugs in Sam. The whole family is freaking out. Did you know he was using?"

"Ted... You knew."

Of course he knew; the three of us had used together. But this was typical of Ted, lying until it became the new truth.

"No, I didn't. Fuck. This all went so wrong."

I didn't know what to say; there was no point in arguing.

"Can I please just come get you? I need to see you."

"I don't want to go to your house," I said. "You can come here. My mom's out."

I regretted those words as soon as I said it. I showered and an hour later he was pulling into the driveway. Our house had a huge arched window in the living room. I watched him get out of the car and could see the invisible tornado around him, the one full of anger and grief and so many red flags. Kasey leaped against the window, barking.

I stood by the front door, holding Kasey by the collar, waiting for Ted to walk up the twenty-eight steps. I think Kasey could see that invisible tornado around Ted, too; he kept growling at him. I ushered Ted up to my room, mainly to keep Kasey from getting agitated. I sat on my bed, next to my wet towel, and looked at my hands in my lap. Ted pushed the balcony door open and went out to have a smoke. I wanted to tell him he couldn't smoke there, but I said nothing. I joined him. There was a slight cool breeze, and it made my neck prickle. Ted began to cry. I put my hand on his back. He cried harder, and I hugged his back. He turned around to kiss me, throwing his cigarette on the Spanish tile roof below us.

"No," I said, pushing him back gently.

He grabbed the back of my head, tenderly at first, and then tightly held my wet hair, pulling me toward his rough mouth.

"Ted, come on."

"Well, haven't you turned into a little bitch," he said as he stormed back inside.

I followed him in. He spun around, grabbed my wrist, and pulled me toward him again, spitting words in my face. "You think you're so fucking special? You're not special. And you're not doing this to me. You hear me?"

Before I could respond, he twisted my body down onto the floor and held me in place while he pulled my leggings down.

"Stop, Ted," I said calmly.

He held me down and kissed my neck, pulled my T-shirt up, and his hands couldn't make up their mind. He got on top of me, pressing the weight of his angry body into me. He pulled my underwear down and pushed his way inside. I didn't fight back. I was paralyzed and, worse, consumed by those old nagging feelings of shame, the kind of shame built on frozen memories. *I am four—his dirty fingernails—don't say anything or I'll kill you, you little slut, you brought this on yourself, hold still, I said hold still.*

I didn't know if I was here or there. I screamed, but no words came out, *This is the same room. This is the same room.*

Suddenly, Ted stopped; he hadn't finished. He pulled his body up and away and collapsed next to me, his head on my chest.

"I'm sorry. I'm sorry. Oh God, Erin, I am so sorry."

My arm hurt; my wrist felt sprained. I just wanted him to leave, so I said, "It's okay. I just want you to leave, though."

And he did. And I didn't speak to him again for years.

After he left, I grabbed my wet towel and got back in the shower. I sat on the floor and gently rubbed my wrist. My neck was sore. After the shower, I called Ellen; I asked her to come to spend the night and she did. I told her that he came over and said he got rough with me—I had to; I had marks on my wrist and throat from his hands—but I didn't tell her about the rape. *Was it rape? Was it like half a rape because he hadn't finished?*

The next week, at my appointment with Dr. Geoffrey, I very much wanted to tell him about what happened with Ted. Instead, I said, "I feel like maybe something happened to me when I was four. But, I don't know, maybe my mind is just making it up."

"Why do you think your mind would make that up?" he asked.

"I don't know."

"What do you think happened?"

"I don't really want to talk about it. Anyway, I think maybe I'm just feeling weird because I saw Ted on Saturday and he's in really bad shape. And he wants me back, but I just don't want that. I feel really guilty about it, though."

"You mention that you feel guilty a lot," Dr. Geoffrey said.

"I do? Well, I mean, I do feel guilty, you know, because I've lied a lot, and I don't know."

"Do you know what all the guilt is really about?" he asked.

"That I've done things I feel guilty about?"

"All that guilt, it's unexpressed anger," he said.

I couldn't respond, but his words clung and multiplied and swarmed around me. I felt my face flush, and I wanted to run out of his office right then and there.

"I don't think I'm angry," I said in a whisper.

"You have a right to be angry, Erin. You have that right."

Dr. Geoffrey's words stayed with me and would come up for me again and again. I would come to see exactly what he meant, that he was right. But after that day, I stopped telling him the whole truth. He listened; he saw me—and I didn't know what to do with that. The attention I used to crave started to scare me. Looking at the truth can be dangerous because behind one truth there are more truths. And one of them is the single thing that you are the most afraid of, the one that's buried underneath years of lies.

If I'd let this go any further, if I let Dr. Geoffrey *know* me, I risked facing trauma I didn't want to face. And worse, what if what he saw was that I was broken, that I was bad? What if at the heart of my anger was a monster, a monster who didn't deserve to be angry, but one who'd caused her own pain all along?

CHAPTER 5
Dazzle
February 1989

I'd settled in well at my new school—a small, liberal Catholic school near the stables and studio lots in Burbank. Ellen and I still spent a lot of time together at school and horseback riding, and I became friends with her friends. I was a sophomore; they were all juniors. I was happier than I'd been in a long time—I had friends, I was off of drugs, and I wasn't miserable over some guy. I'd also returned to professional acting classes, resuming a passion I'd had when I was younger.

Despite all the positive changes, I was still struggling to contain emotional outbursts. I wasn't close enough to my father to feel safe at letting my anger out at him. The worst of this was directed at my mom. I loved her fiercely but also resented her the most. From the time my mom's father had died, when I was four, I couldn't trust which version of her I would get. Sometimes she was distant or depressed, sometimes she was wrapped up in a man, sometimes she was needy and I mothered her. The biggest thorn to me then was that she didn't protect me from the verbal abuse of The Asshole. With him gone and without that opiate buffer that had kept it all suppressed, I found the anger that Dr. Geoffrey had spoken about, the anger I'd denied.

Sometimes, these arguments with my mom escalated to violence. I'd throw things, yell, and physically push her away from me. I had very few rules to follow; when my mom tried to enforce them, I would explode until she backed down. There was a shifting dynamic and I used it to get what I wanted. One afternoon in the kitchen, arguing about something inconsequential, I threw grapes at her and then grabbed a kitchen knife, telling her that I would hurt myself or her if she got any closer.

But the ugliest incident happened one Saturday afternoon when my mom told me I couldn't spend the night at Ellen's, which was an unusual response. Her reasoning was that I spent too many nights away.

"Why doesn't she come here tonight instead?" she asked.

My brain became fixed, in that hormonal teenage way, on getting what I wanted. My mom followed me around the house as I gathered my things and prepared to leave anyway. All I knew was that I wanted out—out of that house, away from her, away from all the resentment I felt. She was close behind me as I made my way around the dining room to the kitchen. I stopped, picked up a dining room chair, and threw it at her. She fell to the floor, crying. *What have I done?* I was sick on anger; I couldn't stop myself even though this wasn't who I wanted to be.

At Dr. Geoffrey's urging, I started having sessions with each of my parents. My mom was also in therapy. One afternoon, after school, we sat in the sanctuary of Dr. Geoffrey's office. My mom and I sat on opposite ends of a big leather sofa. I slouched, leaning my body as far away as possible. My mom was tearing up and picking at a tissue in her hands before we even started.

"Why don't you tell me how things have been at home lately," Dr. Geoffrey said to my mom.

My mom let out a deep sigh and said, "I'm scared of her. I…"

I rolled my eyes and let out my own sigh of irritation.

She turned toward me. "I am, Erin." And she turned back to Dr. Geoffrey. "Did she tell you she threw a chair at me? It left a mark."

"Where do you think this anger is coming from?" he asked, directing the question at her.

"I don't know," she said.

Dr. Geoffrey turned toward me, and I felt stinging hot tears that I was desperate to contain. "Erin, can you try to explain to your mom where some of this anger might be coming from?"

"You want to know why I'm angry? Let's start with the fact that she had some asshole living with us who was so mean to me and she just let it happen."

I turned toward my mom and continued, "You always chose him first! Always! And he doesn't even love you. He hated me. And you let him hate me."

I continued on like this for several minutes that felt like one long hot red moment that had trapped us all. When I was done, I could see my mom struggling to keep herself together through deep, heaving sobs. And I felt guilty again.

She took a moment and said, looking at Dr. Geoffrey, "I am so sorry." Then turned to me and repeated, "I am so, so sorry, Erin. You're right. I didn't protect you from him. I can imagine how awful that felt. I am so sorry."

I can't emphasize enough how important it was for me to hear those words from her, to hear them without any *but*s attached. It was the first time I'd felt validated in so long. Still, I didn't feel safe enough with her, with anyone really, to tell her *everything*. Much like pushing away the unclear memories I had from when I was four, I felt a frenzied need to shield the people closest to me from the truth, from the truths about me that would make them look at me differently. At the heart of all these things that happened, I felt culpable. If they were my fault, I had some control over them. *I* was the monster. That felt less scary, although over time being the monster would come to feel more terrifying. But then, as a teenager, those secrets made me feel safe, or safer.

After that session, I didn't tell her about the drugs or the rape, but I did tell her that I'd lost a friend the year before and that I'd had a boyfriend I never told her about. In turn, she opened up to me about her teenage years—about her first boyfriend when her family lived in Japan, about her father's volatility and mother's silence, and about the time her father beat her so severely she thought he was going to kill her. It shocked me, but it made some of the ways she acted make more sense—like freezing up when The Asshole got angry, like cowering on the floor when I threw the chair at her. Maybe we were not so different—we both held secrets, some we shared and some we held close. But the therapy and what we did open up about improved our relationship, at least for a while.

My dad came to a couple of therapy sessions with me. They were wholly unproductive and mostly devolved into talking about my mom and her problems. My dad was in LA frequently, or at least at his beach house, but I had little interest in spending time with him. We both held each other at a distance and I couldn't bear to change that. I already felt like he didn't really like me—and that was the me I *let* him see. If I let him get any closer, I'd know for sure he didn't love me. That was the root of my relationship with him; I was so afraid he didn't love me. The only tangible proof I had of his affection were things, things he bought me over the years—toys and vacations and dinners and clothes, then horses and acting classes and money to go shopping.

My best memories with my dad were when I would visit him in New York. I loved New York City. I felt like I belonged there. LA never felt like home—all that sunny sameness coating everything. New York City was an explosion of art and music and museums and theater and restaurants and glamour.

While my dad was at work, he would give me cash and his Amex, with a note giving me permission to use his card. That action—that monetary exchange—made me feel protected and provided for. I think about this now as a parent and I understand his motivation. As a parent there can be an overwhelming desire to fix things for your kid, to erase their sadness and pain. Although my dad didn't know the extent of what was happening with me, I believe he sensed it and this was the only way he knew to *fix* it.

On those days—cash and Amex in tow—I'd go shopping and almost always end my day with tea at The Plaza, in The Palm Court. I loved it there—all that green and gold, and tea and scones with clotted cream, and tiny sandwiches, strawberries and whipped cream, and the violinist and piano player, sometimes a harp. When I was done, I'd wait outside, in front of the Paris Theatre, for my dad to meet me. We'd often head down to TKTS for half-price show tickets and always dinner.

My father seemed to enjoy his single life in New York, and when I'd visit he would take me out with him and his wingman, a younger guy who worked with him. We'd go to China Club or Monkey Bar, and I'd never get carded. Of course, I'd spend my night pretending I wasn't there with my dad, but a grown adult living in NYC. It was fun, but it was all surface. It was all small talk and chatter and a turnstile of new people to meet.

Back home in LA, Ellen and I had a new obsession—boys in bands. It was the end of an era on the Sunset Strip. Glam rock bands were still around, but grunge was about to take over. On a typical Friday and Saturday night, Ellen and I, along with other friends, would descend upon the Sunset Strip. We'd park and spend a couple of hours walking up and down the north side of Sunset between San Vicente and Doheny, past the Whiskey-A-Go-Go, The Roxy and The Rainbow Room, and Gazzarri's. It was a sea of guys and girls in heavy makeup and hair spray and latex clothing. We'd flirt and talk to the guys passing out gig flyers. As the clubs closed and people poured out onto the sidewalks headed to after-parties, we'd end up at

Pennyfeather's on La Cienega, where we'd be almost certain to see Rodney Bingenheimer sitting alone at a table, happily striking up conversations with us, or Rock 'n' Roll Denny's on Sunset near Fairfax, which was always filled up with bikers and glam rockers.

We didn't have IDs to get into these various clubs unless it was on an all-ages night, until another friend from school, who was the grandson of one of the club owners, got us fake birth certificates. This was when Marisol Marissa Glass was born. I was fifteen; she was eighteen. Because this was the dark ages, before everything was computerized, all it took was my thumbprint and that fake piece of paper. I've often wondered if somehow my thumbprint still exists in old DMV records under two names.

That fake ID allowed us entry to a whole new world of clubs and older guys and excitement but, most important, the music. I had always loved music, loved seeking out indie bands as well as classic stuff like old Bowie and T. Rex, Roxy Music and The Velvet Underground. But being able to see live music—that was life changing. On the occasional school night that we were allowed to go out, we'd dance away at Club 1970 or English Acid. And through all those late nights and boys and bands, I didn't touch any drugs or alcohol. I'd even stopped stealing pills from people's medicine cabinets.

In mid-February, I went with a group of friends to see the local bands Pretty Boy Floyd and The Zeros at The Roxy. As we stood in the very crowded club, I felt someone's eyes on me. I looked around and saw a guy who resembled a glammed-out Johnny Depp crossed with Sid Vicious staring back at me. He had long black hair, wore way more eyeliner than I did, and had an energy that felt all at once familiar and brand-new; my heart stopped. I couldn't quite identify the feeling I was having—*was it déjà vu; was it love at first sight?* We didn't speak, and I didn't see him again for months, but I didn't forget him.

Later that summer, Ellen and I ran smack-dab into him on the Sunset Strip, where he was handing out flyers for his band. Ian and I became friends instantly. He was eighteen, had moved here with his band from Las Vegas, and was living in a rehearsal space above Hollywood Billiards. He made my stomach drop every time I saw him, but I did my best to act real casual. We hung out with my friends and his, at clubs, on the Strip, and sometimes in his band's rehearsal space and home.

By fall of 1989, I accepted that we were deep in the "friend zone," but I spoke about him incessantly to my girlfriends. At school, we passed notes back and forth in a spiral-bound notebook, detailing our fantasies of dating, kissing, and living happily ever after with various guys from the local music scene. Increasingly, the only one I dreamed about was Ian. Somehow, for the first time in a long time, I felt like other girls my age—boy crazy, not hiding a closet full of drugs and sex and secrets. I'd even told my mom about Ian.

About a month before my sixteenth birthday, my dad was in town and took Ellen and me to look at cars. I had my heart set on a Jeep Cherokee. We hadn't set out to buy a car that day, just to look. But that Saturday evening, there we were seated in the Jeep dealership talking price. My dad had a date back at the beach and the clock was ticking. He ended up writing a check and suddenly I had a brand-new car. This was another instance of my dad showing his affection—through the buying of things—and I happily accepted.

I wasn't sixteen and hadn't even made the appointment to get my driver's license yet. Ellen drove us back to her house and my dad headed off to his date, a hero in my eyes, at least for that night. When we got to Ellen's, I called my mom to share the good news. She was furious at my father for making that decision without her. She thought it was extravagant, and she was right. But at the time, her reaction pissed me off.

My sixteenth birthday came and went. About a week after my

birthday, we ran into Ian at English Acid. Ian was in a corner whispering with Shelly, a mutual friend, and I felt sick. *What are they talking about? He probably likes her.* I wanted to leave. They finished their conversation, and he disappeared. Shelly grabbed me by the hand, and we serpentined through the small rooms of English Acid, '70s glam rock blaring, old videos of Sweet and Gary Glitter projected on the walls.

We found Ian hanging out alone, seated in one of the back rooms. Shelly grabbed his hand, yanked him up, and said, "Enough of this crap. Erin, he's totally in love with you. Ian, she adores you. Talk to each other." And my heart opened up for the very first time.

I fell for Ian with an innocence and abandon that had been missing with Ted. I'd pick him up; we'd drive around, listen to music, make out. But he wouldn't have sex with me. He was hung up on the fact that I was only sixteen. At first, it made things seem magical, like I'd never done those things with anyone before. We spent countless nights holding hands, electricity tying us together—whispering, laughing, kissing until our lips were blistered. I told him everything about Ted and the drugs and the lies I'd kept as a barrier between me and just about everyone. Ian didn't drink or do drugs; both of his parents were alcoholics, and his grandparents raised him. He made me feel safe and seen and heard. I thought we were invincible.

The one person not thrilled by my new relationship was Ellen. All the nights I used to spend with Ellen were now reserved for Ian. I couldn't go riding on a Saturday afternoon because I was going to watch his band practice. Sleepovers with frozen yogurt and rented movies? Sorry, hanging out with Ian. I'd meet her at the club instead of riding there with her.

As 1989 tipped into 1990, Ellen broke up with me. She gave me an ultimatum. She didn't exactly ask me to break up with him, but she made it clear that I either stopped neglecting our friendship or we wouldn't be friends at all. I was livid. *Here I am, finally happy, and she's trying to ruin it.* But she was right; I was neglecting our friendship. On a Sunday afternoon in early January, Ellen stopped by to drop off my things and pick up hers. We stood on the top landing, outside my front door.

"Well, I guess this is it," she said.

"Yup. I guess so."

"I really hope that you're happy."

"I am," I said defensively. I wanted to say, *Don't go. I'll be a better friend. I promise.* Instead I watched her walk away. And just like that, I'd lost my best friend. I was devastated, and I didn't want to lose Ian, too, and that made me cling to him even more.

In late January, I got into a car accident with a wall, thanks to my novice driving skills, and I suddenly found myself carless and would be for three months. Not having a car impacted my relationship with Ian; we weren't able to see each other as frequently. I forged new friendships. One of these was with Lila, whom I'd met through another girl at school. Lila was like a teenage Elvira—busty with porcelain skin and long black hair. She lived close by, and we spent more and more time together—having sleepovers (usually at her house) and going out to clubs like death rock mecca Helter Skelter. We both had divorced parents and our moms formed a friendship, too. Lila became like a sister to me and remains one of my best friends today.

I began to focus more on acting and less on horses. A back injury made riding every day and competing much less appealing. I also found out that I could graduate early, at the end of my junior year. My social life both at school and outside school was thriving, but something was amiss. As spring arrived, Ian was pulling away.

In May, we went a week without talking. He wouldn't return my calls. I heard from his bandmate that he'd gone out of town with another girl—not a girl, a woman—also named Erin. I refused to believe it. When he got back, he called me and said we needed to talk. When I got to the house he shared with his bandmates, he was waiting outside for me. He climbed inside my car and I killed the engine. He couldn't look me in the eye. He just stared at his hands in his lap.

"I don't think we should see each other for a while," he said, fixated on his hands.

"What do you mean? Why?"

"I'm no good for you, Erin. You're sixteen. You should be focusing on school and dating someone your own age."

"Are you kidding me right now? I'm not an idiot. I know you're seeing someone else."

"This isn't about anyone else," he said, but he didn't deny it. "Erin, I love you so much, more than I've ever loved anyone. It's just not good timing. And I don't want you to hate me. I'd die if you hated me."

"Well, then, I guess you're dead because I fucking hate you."

We sat in silence for what seemed like an eternity.

"Just get out of my car."

Ian opened the car door, pausing for a minute, taking a deep breath, and said, "I do love you. I always will."

And with that, he was gone.

It was a searing rejection. I didn't believe him. *The age thing is an excuse. He doesn't love you. You're stupid and ugly. How could he love you?* This was the first time I'd felt this sort of heartbreak, the kind that leaves traces behind in your skin for future lovers to find. I drove home, sobbing, aching, devastated.

In that final month of school, I shuffled through my days, sullen and broken. I listened to Sinead O'Connor sing "Nothing Compares 2 U" over and over. At home, I watched *Sid & Nancy* on repeat, unable to sleep most nights. And I started stealing pills again.

Once summer was in full swing, I spent almost every night at a club—Club 1970, English Acid, Helter Skelter, Kontrol Faktory, Club Fuck, Jabberjaw. I found myself falling into old drug habits, although I swore to myself I would never touch heroin again. Instead, it was crystal meth and pills. And men. I wanted casual sex, no strings, constant validation. As a sixteen-year-old, that wasn't hard to come by.

Ian and I ran into each other from time to time, and it was always awkward at best, painful and hostile at worst. One night in July, he confronted me. He knew I was using; he called me out on it immediately, adding that it hurt him to see me let lecherous guys "hang all over me." I quickly reminded him that what I did or who I did it with was none of his business. A week later, I was shocked to see him out at a club, drunk. We were both spinning out of control, in opposite directions, and for that I blamed him.

CHAPTER 6

Superstition
1991–1993

"Do you like kiwi?" my Persian grandmother asked in her squeaky voice, presenting me with a small plate of delicately sliced rounds of bright green kiwi.

It was her eighth going on eightieth attempt at getting me to eat something on a hot Saturday afternoon in May of 1991. I was there at her house—a ten-minute drive from my mom's—to see my dad, who was in town for the weekend. Persian Grandma looked and sounded a bit like Dr. Ruth and her main objective was to get the people she loved to eat. She was relentless. We weren't close, not like I was with my maternal grandmother, but she was bright and determined with showing her affection. Persian food was and still is a source of comfort and familiarity for me, but in those days, I was more concerned with crystal meth and *not* eating, and the last thing in the world I felt like on a hot Saturday afternoon were my childhood favorites—*tadig* and *fesenjoon*.

Dad and I sat opposite each other in her living room, as my grandmother continued to pile things on plates and offer them up. My dad was half listening to me as I was making a case for getting an apartment instead of living in a dorm at USC. My dad was always distracted, always seeming to look beyond me on to the next boating trip or the next date he had or something work related, which made me feel small and unimportant. For as long as I could remember and for many, many years to come, the only way I *felt* any love from him was when he was buying me something. And I had become hell-bent on getting what I wanted—toys, a horse, another horse, a car, money for clothes, an apartment, travel. I would cajole and pester and sometimes manipulate until I got my way. I knew it was wrong to "work" him the way I did and each time I got something, it added to my sense of guilt, as if he didn't really want me to have the object.

Oh, you didn't get that thing? Well, see, he doesn't love you. And, oh, sure, you got a toy/car/horse/money and you don't deserve it, you stupid piece of shit, spoiled brat. Every time you take that money, that thing you don't deserve, you get closer to being the piece of shit you really are. Look at how many people don't have anything, anything at all, and here you are, on your knees, asking for more and more. You spoiled bitch.

"So, like I was saying, I looked at this apartment in Hollywood, like, north of Franklin, off of Vine. It's basically Beachwood Canyon. But I would have to put a deposit down on it now. I just really think it would be better for me to not live with Mom anymore. And a dorm? I don't know. It's not really safe down at USC, you know? Do you think we could go look at the place today?"

He was nodding his head, but I could tell he hadn't heard a word.

"Mâmân," he said, and with that, he left me dangling and started speaking to his mother in Farsi, a language I did not speak, before getting up and leaving the room.

I walked outside and sat on the doorstep. There was something about my dad not listening that made me feel desperate. Waves of heat rippled over me. He eventually opened the front door and saw me sitting there.

"What are you doing?" he asked.

"You weren't listening."

"I was listening...so what did you say?" he said and chuckled.

I could feel my face get hot, flustered by his dismissal. He wasn't being mean; this was and still is my dad's sense of humor. But to my teenage brain, it felt like an insult, like a cherry on top of years of not paying attention to me.

"If you don't get me my own apartment, I'll start stripping," I said in an egregious attempt at manipulation, and my ears started to ring.

"Erin, don't be ridiculous..." He went into some sort of lecture.

The ringing in my ears got louder, and I couldn't hear the words coming out of his mouth. *He doesn't love you, run, run, run,* crashed around in between my ears. A sharp tingling started in my fingertips and quickly swept up my arms. I had to get out of there.

I ran to my car and sped away. On the short drive to my mom's, my arms felt paralyzed. I wondered if I might crash. I thought about what it would feel like if I did, that moment of impact and metal and glass and my body pressing all together. I was hyperventilating, but not loudly or in a way that was obvious. I'd just stopped breathing, my body unable to bring in oxygen.

When I got home, my mom was waiting for me. My dad had called and told her I had a freak-out. She tried to talk to me about it, but I resisted. And to her credit, she understood. She knew how my dad could be dismissive with a look or a word or lack of words, and how that could make you feel so very, very small.

Dave, my mom's new boyfriend, was there, too. I liked Dave. He was the epitome of a laid-back, tan, blond Californian— good-looking in a Don Johnson sort of way. That afternoon, Dave sat with me and listened. He validated my feelings. He understood panic attacks; he'd long dealt with them, too. He knew what it was to have the paralysis of anxiety grip you and shake you and not let go. He *saw* me.

During the course of his relationship with my mom, he would have conversations like this with me many, many times. I will always be grateful for the person he was to me in my life then. In many ways, he showed up as the father figure I needed, the kind my dad was just not capable of being.

I drove back to my grandmother's after I had calmed down. My dad made a joke about my speedy exit, and we left it at that. I didn't tell him what I needed from him, wanted from him emotionally, because I didn't believe I would ever get it.

What I did get was my own apartment. I was still a minor, but the management company allowed it, as my two roommates were over eighteen, and my dad cosigned for us all. My first apartment was on the first floor of a renovated old classic Hollywood building on Franklin just west of Western Avenue. It had a nice lobby and a live-in super. The long, carpeted hallways conjured images of *The Shining*. It was a two-bedroom, one bath. I had the "master," one roommate had the second bedroom, and the other turned the dining nook into her bedroom, cordoned off by a folding screen we bought at Pier One Imports. We moved in July of 1991. By November, we had a mold problem. By December, we had a mold problem and roommate squabbles. By January, we were in the process of breaking our lease and moving out.

"Eh-eh."

I cringed at the sound of Mike-Jim clearing his throat as I lay next to him, back to back, in my queen-size bed, my forehead resting on the wall. I studied the stucco wall in front of me. *Is that mold along the baseboard again? Ugh.* I called him Mike-Jim because he went by Mike, but his name was Jim, or the other way around. Frankly, I don't think either was his real name.

The thing I remember most about Mike-Jim was his incessant throat clearing. Sometimes it was an "eh-eh," and sometimes it was a "glech-huh." And he did it all the time. When I asked him about it, he laughed like I was making it up. I wasn't making it up.

I should also probably tell you the other thing about Mike-Jim. He was a drug dealer—mostly crystal meth, some ecstasy, a little bit of weed, and occasionally pills. Mike-Jim's signature look was death rock surfer. My attraction to Mike-Jim was 2 percent his skinny boy body, floppy blond hair, and devilish grin, and 98 percent access to my drug of choice du jour—crystal meth.

On that Saturday morning in January of 1992, Mike-Jim had spent the night—*for two weeks*. I hadn't realized on our first date that he didn't technically live anywhere. That afternoon, I drove Mike-Jim to an unassuming apartment at the bottom of Beachwood Canyon to pick up drugs from his supplier. Mike-Jim knocked on the screen door, clearing his throat. A tall, skinny guy with long dark hair who looked like he walked straight out of casting for a Lynyrd Skynyrd biopic answered the door.

"Come on in," he said with a slight drawl. "I'm Bill."

He stuck out his hand and shook mine, then pointed to the leather couch in the sparsely furnished apartment. "Sit down."

Bill walked to the kitchen and came back, put a can of Coke on the glass coffee table in front of me, and nodded at me.

"Thanks," I said.

I sat on the edge of the couch and smiled politely, watching as Bill weighed plum-size rocks of crystal meth on a scale before placing them in Tupperware containers that Mike-Jim put into his large metal briefcase. When they were done, Bill and Mike-Jim went into the corner and talked in hushed tones. Mike-Jim handed him a wad of cash. He turned to me and signaled that I should get up.

"Nice to meet you, and thanks for the Coke," I said to Bill, who nodded, humming.

Mike-Jim was not great at being a drug dealer. For starters, he got high on his own supply. And when he did, he gave away drugs to people like me. Later that night we went to a going-away party for Lila, who was heading to England for a semester abroad. Mike-Jim brought the drugs. But he also brought his personality and his throat clearing and his excessive talking about his ex-girlfriend. After the party, I told him that he could spend one last night at my place, but after that, he should stay somewhere else.

The next day, I dropped him off in the Valley, at the home of some random relative of his in Calabasas. He asked me to hold on to the metal briefcase because he "couldn't bring drugs into that house." When I got back to my apartment, I opened up the briefcase, opened up the Tupperware containers, and broke off little rocks of crystal meth, putting them into several small plastic bags. I took one small rock, crushed it with the back of a credit card onto my textbook for Introduction to Neuroscience, and proceeded to chop it, forming three small lines, which I snorted up with a piece of small straw from my McDonald's Coke.

The powder burned, filling my nostrils with a smell specific to methamphetamines. The scent is decidedly and expectedly chemical, sort of like Clorox, with a very faint undertone of fake flowers. I closed my eyes, gritted my teeth, and took a few sharp breaths as the speedy rush amped up my heart rate. Crystal put me in what I like to call the artificial up. It's not as gregarious as cocaine. It's sort of manageable if you control the amount you use. It always made me feel alert, precise, and wholly compartmentalized. It didn't quite offer me the same disconnect that heroin did, but since I'd made a promise to myself to stay away from heroin, it became a convenient substitute.

I pressed the containers shut, put them back in the briefcase, and wondered where I should store the thing. I have made some questionable decisions in my life. The decision to store the drugs in the trunk of my Jetta is right up there with the poorest, most cringe-worthy decisions I've ever made.

Some might say it's a miracle that I never got pulled over, never got caught with that briefcase of drugs. But I see it less as a miracle and more because I was a young woman with passing-white privilege in a Jetta. I've thought about this often, that had my skin been darker, had I come from less privilege, I have no doubt that I would have been arrested early on. I've thought about how that would have changed the trajectory of my life, how early arrests might have kept me forever trapped in a cycle of incarceration. Our drug laws are undeniably skewed to keep people of color and people of less privilege imprisoned and enslaved. And I've always been aware of that.

As fun as it was to be able to break off tiny rocks whenever the mood struck me, which was happening every day, I knew that no good could come of this kind of access. Finally, after two weeks, I drove that briefcase in my trunk out to another house in Calabasas.

"Eh-eh, thanks, glech-huh. I'll call you," he said as I skipped down the driveway.

I never saw Mike-Jim again or heard another word from him.

In February, I moved into a charming Spanish-style one-bedroom on Los Feliz Boulevard, and I started dating Will. I was now eighteen, and Will was twenty-six. He was soft-spoken, polite, and handsome—tall and pale with dark brown hair and large puppy-dog eyes—and he counted inventory for pharmacies by day and made music on keyboards at night. After a couple of months, we made the brilliant (read: stupid) decision to move in together. I'd stopped using crystal meth and was only, occasionally, taking pills. Will would sometimes pocket a tablet or two while doing inventory, and much as in past relationships, the access to drugs he provided was a bonus for me.

My relationship with Will was toxic, and I was the one who brought the toxicity. I treated him unkindly, I made out with other guys and lied about it, and I threw tantrums—literal tantrums, throwing objects, pounding my fists on the floor, embarrassing tantrums—when I felt he wasn't giving me enough attention, or conversely when I felt smothered. To be Will in a relationship with me could not have been fun. And inevitably, there was a breaking point.

Ten months into our relationship, in January of 1993, I went to San Francisco on a girls' trip with Lila and her Scottish girlfriend she'd met during her semester abroad. We arrived back in Los Angeles on a rainy Sunday evening. When I walked in the door of my apartment, my mom was there, seated in the living room with Will. I was confused. They both seemed nervous. I looked around and noticed that the room looked different, like things were missing. And they were.

"What's going on?" I asked, finally, to break the awkward silence.

"Can we go in the bedroom and talk?" Will asked.

I looked at my mom, and she gave me a half smile and looked down. *What's going on?*

Will sat me on the bed and told me in one very long run-on sentence that he was leaving me, he had moved all of his things out, he would be moving to San Francisco in two weeks, and he was sorry. I was blindsided, and my ego took the wheel. I threw things at him, hit him, threatened to kill myself. I ran to the kitchen and grabbed a knife. I did and said many things that filled me with humiliation the next morning. I was a two-year-old in the body of a nineteen-year-old. My mom calmed me down, convinced me to go spend the night at her house. He was smart to have asked her to be there, but it stung to learn that my mom knew about my breakup before I did.

In the weeks that followed, I continued the drama. I was trying to convince myself that I loved him, that we belonged together. What I was actually reeling from was the rejection; the rejection meant he saw all the things in me that I was sure made me unlovable. *He knows I'm a monster.* I became determined to win him back. I thought about moving to San Francisco. I cried on couches—Lila's and my old roommates'. I slept on my friends Polly and Milo's bedroom floor, next to their bed because I was afraid to be alone. They were all good friends and exceedingly patient with me.

One night, about six weeks after we'd broken up, I was on the phone with Will and I told him of my very determined plan to move to San Francisco. He stopped me midsentence.

"Erin, I really don't think it's a good idea for you to move here. Or for us to talk. Because if we do, if we keep talking, we'll probably get back together and that scares me."

"I know I wasn't easy, Will. But I'm not the same person I was."

"No, you don't get it," he replied. "I'm afraid I might kill you."

I laughed. We sat in silence; it took me a moment to process what he meant. "Kill me? What do you mean, kill me?" I asked.

"Do you remember a couple weeks before we broke up, you got really sick off of that spaghetti?"

"The food poisoning?" I asked.

"It wasn't food poisoning."

"What do you mean?"

"I put thirty phenobarbitals in your spaghetti," he said casually.

"What? I don't understand."

"I stole some phenobarbitals, and I don't know. I was mad."

"You were mad?" I asked.

"Yeah. The night before, when you went to James's, I spied on you. I saw you. You made out with him."

I was stunned. "Wait, you saw me?"

"I looked through his side window."

"From the bushes?"

"Yes. But whatever. Really, I just wanted you to not fucking talk. I didn't want to hear one more lying word come out of your mouth. And I'm afraid that I could do something like that again."

"Wow," I said. "Yeah, I think we should probably call it a day."

With that, I hung up the phone, and I never saw or spoke to Will again. It was miraculous; all the pining and hurt and desperation born of rejection disappeared. His revelation was the slap I needed to snap out of my fixation on winning him back. And incidentally, I think it might have been my pill tolerance that saved me from the botched spaghetti poisoning. I never reported it. I wanted to be done with that chapter, and I was. It was much easier to turn it into a funny anecdote—*hey, did I ever tell you about the time I got poisoned*—rather than face the reality that the man I lived with, who said he loved me, tried to kill me. How I handled that truth from Will is how I increasingly handled everything in my life—*compartmentalize, shrug off, minimize, laugh about, put away in a box that you shove in a closet and never look at again.*

Shortly after that call with Will, I began an affair with a significantly older married man—a somewhat famous, short, Irish singer who liked to hit me during sex. I couldn't decide if I liked it or hated it. He seduced me over long dinners soaked with red wine and Leonard Cohen. We talked about books and film and philosophy. The intellectual stimulation was stronger than I'd had before from a relationship. He had just moved to LA, getting ready to put out a new album and prepare for a US tour. The fact that he was married was like an insurance policy for me. I knew going in what I would get, and that kept me from getting hurt. I was becoming more adept at this compartmentalization thing, not knowing how it would affect me long-term.

By summer, I started dating Brett, someone I'd been friends with for a while. Brett was hilarious and whip-smart; he was a few inches shorter than me and he reminded me of Ethan Hawke in *Reality Bites*. Our friend groups overlapped, and my life was feeling stable—I was taking pills infrequently and getting along with my parents when I saw them. But a change of seasons was coming.

★ ★ ★

Brett and I were playing pool with Polly and Milo at a cof-feehouse on Franklin, at the base of the Hollywood Hills, that was like our Central Perk. I went outside to have a cigarette, a new habit I had begun indulging. As I stood next to the news-stand on the side street in the mild late-September air, I looked across the street at a house that I recognized. It belonged to old family friends of my parents. A man dragged a trash can to the curb, and the streetlight lit up his face. I knew the contours of that face—the sharp cheekbones and pronounced jaw and the shape of his head and his mouth. He was the son of those friends, now an adult.

A cold sweat coated my body; I couldn't move. I stopped breathing. I knew. *I fucking knew.* I could finally identify what that nagging feeling had been all those years in the pit of my stomach—the one that filled me with shame, the one that made me a monster. It was *him.* It was his angry adolescent fingers that had pushed their way inside me when I was four, when I was five, when I was six—*how many times?* It was the sneer on his face when he tore my bathing suit off when I was twelve, pushing my head underwater in the swimming pool of family friends. It was the rage he'd infected me with that I'd turned into shame and guilt and self-loathing. A flood of recall poured through my cells. I began to hyperventilate.

The feelings, the moments, the sounds, the touch—everything came back, but all out of order. That's the thing about trauma; it disperses bits and pieces of information and hands them back to you like an undone jigsaw puzzle. It can take hours or days or weeks or years or a lifetime to put them all together in the right place, the right order. And I'm sure that's what saves us. I'm sure that's what helps us get up the next morning and the morning after that, because having it all together, all lined up, it's just too much. But that disorder is also what makes us doubt things, for years.

I sat on the curb and put my head down. I felt like I was going to pass out. Polly came out to find me. She knelt down and put her hand on my forehead.

"Erin, what's going on?" she asked.

Polly's long red hair and Kewpie doll face were a welcome sight. I grabbed her hand and pulled her to sit down next to me.

"What is it?" she asked.

I couldn't speak.

"It's okay. Just breathe. Take a deep breath in through your nose. Good. And out through your mouth."

Once she had me breathing more or less, she ran back inside to get Brett and Milo. Back at my apartment, once I'd calmed down, I told them what happened. I told them who he was and what he'd done and what I remembered in all its scattered bits and pieces. I told them how he'd pin me down on my six-foot-tall stuffed dog, Henry, and he'd scratch me and breathe right on me and tell me that he'd kill me if I said anything and that no one would believe me.

Brett and Polly were solidly supportive. They listened and didn't try to fix it, and at that moment that was all I needed. I later told Lila about it as well. It felt like I was making a breakthrough; I remembered and was talking about it.

But then, as quickly as that door to possible healing opened, it shut again. I stopped wanting to talk about it. I wish I could point to why or how that happened, but I can't. I wasn't able to do anything more with that trauma. I started looking through medicine cabinets again, taking pills again.

"But I'm fine. Really, I'm fine now," I told them.

And somehow, they believed me.

CHAPTER 7
Passages
November 1993

Two months after I'd seen him—after all those memories descended on me like shrapnel—I shifted parts of my life again in an effort to keep moving. I needed to keep pushing forward, and somehow leave those wounds behind me. I took a leave of absence from school; I wanted to pursue acting, as I had when I was younger. I enrolled in a professional acting class and got a part-time job at a well-known and popular boutique in Hollywood. I chopped my long hair off into a Louise Brooks–style bob. I wanted to reinvent myself. I wanted to distance myself from the person I was, the one who had been carrying pain and shame and running from it in vain, faster and faster.

Brett was a loyal and caring boyfriend, but after that September evening outside the coffeehouse, I felt suffocated by his tenderness. I began to recognize, at least peripherally, that anytime emotional intimacy was developing, in both romantic and platonic relationships, I would shut down. As much as I longed to be seen and heard and cared for, I couldn't bear it; being close to someone was dangerous. I had a tendency to push people away when I'd revealed too much. I told Brett I wanted an open re-lationship, and he reluctantly agreed.

In early November, I was standing behind the front counter at work, wearing one of the shop's signature navy-and-maroon-striped French aprons, on a quiet Tuesday afternoon. A famous actor—let's call him Keith—walked in and asked if he could leave his motorcycle helmet behind the counter. He was tall and handsome, with chiseled features, soulful eyes, and messy hair. He had that just-rolled-out-of-bed quality and emitted a subtle sexual energy. Having grown up in LA, I thought nothing of it; the boutique was frequented by a lot of celebrities. On his way out, he made small talk with me—told me he liked my hair-cut and we talked about PJ Harvey. The thing that struck me about him was an almost imperceptible sadness, like the kind I had, the kind that people hide underneath fame and money and drugs and sex. About an hour after he left, he called the store and asked to speak with me.

"Hey, I'm the guy with the motorcycle helmet," he said, as if that was what made him memorable and not the dozen films I'd seen him in.

"Hey, how's it going?"

"I wanted to ask for your number and see what you're doing later tonight," he said.

"Well, um, I can give you my number, but you should know I have a boyfriend."

We met up the next night at a coffeehouse near the boutique that was full of velvet couches and little wooden tables. During our coffee date, I learned he was mourning the loss of a friend and he had a complicated family history. We loved a lot of the same bands, and he really liked my hair, which he touched hesitantly with his hand, brushing my bangs aside. It was awk-ward but also endearing. I should have wanted him. There were scores of girls my age who would have loved to be in my shoes, but there was something that stopped me from letting him in, at least all the way. I felt suspicious of him. I felt suspicious of most men, particularly the ones who wanted something from me. *How could he want me? Can't he see I'm rotten?*

After coffee, we stood in the alley behind the coffeehouse and he kissed me. And he was a damn good kisser, an intuitive kisser. His kisses were confident but not pushy. He pulled back from me, and put his hand on the back of my hair, stroking my head and looking at me. It made me so uncomfortable.

"When can I see you again?" he asked.

"You know I have a boyfriend."

"Then what are you doing here?"

"I don't know. I mean I'm allowed to date other people, but, like, this can't be a serious thing."

"Is that so…" He smiled and I could tell he didn't believe me.

This was all too familiar. I repeatedly found myself in situations with men who wanted a piece of me. They wanted more than sex; they wanted emotional intimacy. Like an anorexic with food, I would cut myself off from my feelings. I was back in control. And the more I withheld, the more the men in my life wanted in. I withheld sex, I withheld affection, I withheld "I like you" and "I love you."

Withholding was my new drug.

This affected Keith worst of all. His mental health was in a precarious place as it was. He had been grappling with depression and anxiety and was conflicted about his increasing fame. We'd developed a terrible pattern of flirting, sometimes kissing, sometimes fooling around, and me always pulling back and pushing him away. I kept him in murky territory, giving him just enough to want more but not enough to ever feel seen or wanted or loved. Brett, meanwhile, began pulling away from me. We should have broken up; we were living separate lives— both playing games and no one was winning.

In addition to Keith and Brett, I continued to casually date other guys. It was remarkable how not wanting anything made men want everything. I felt like I'd figured out the secret to never getting hurt again.

My lease was up on my apartment, and in February of 1994, I moved in with Polly and Milo, as their roommate had just moved out. The apartment was in Beachwood Canyon, a couple of blocks north of drug dealer Bill's place, where I'd gone with Mike-Jim.

Keith was renting a house up near the Hollywood sign and would ride past my apartment on his motorcycle, going up and down the canyon. He was also dabbling with drugs, and his behavior got erratic. Sometimes, he'd stop and throw pebbles at my bedroom window, which faced the street, or he'd call in the middle of the night, send flowers to my work, to my apartment. He followed me and had me followed when I was out with Brett.

Despite all this, I was never afraid of Keith; I never felt like he would harm me. He had fame and money and there were countless women who wanted him, but he was lost. I understood that type of lost. He was looking for something in me that I was unwilling—no, unable—to give him, and I resented him for that because I felt he saw something in me, something special, that just didn't exist.

One night, Polly came home with news. Ian, the first one who broke my heart, got married. This hit me unexpectedly hard; it pushed me and Ian even further away from a possible reconciliation, something I'd secretly and foolishly held on to. But there was more. He was sick, really sick. The drinking that had started after we broke up had taken a giant toll in four short years.

I called Keith and asked him to pick me up. He did. We rode down Sunset on his motorcycle and went to the Chateau Marmont, where he stayed from time to time. I sat on the edge of the king-size bed in his airy white hotel room. The door to the balcony was open, letting in a moist breeze. My hands were shaking. I couldn't feel my fingers. He sat down next to me and took hold of my shaky hands.

"Your hands are so cold," he said, kissing my fingertips.

"I'll be right back," I said.

Back in another bathroom, I sat on the floor and fumbled in my purse for an Altoids tin. When I found it, I opened it up and poured the contents—four Vicodin—into my hand. I stood up, filled a glass with water from the sink, and swallowed the pills.

"Can we watch a movie?" I asked, settling myself in, back on the bed.

Keith put on *The Age of Innocence*. We propped ourselves up on pillows at the foot of the bed and lay on our stomachs, feet against the headboard. As the Vicodin began to work its way into my bloodstream, a warm fuzzy ring formed around me. I looked at Keith. He looked at me.

"Are you feeling any better?" he asked.

"Can you hold me?" I shocked myself asking that. I usually hated being held; I found it suffocating.

Before he could answer, I took off my clothes and got under the covers. He got into bed with me, pulled me toward him, and brought my head into his warm chest, and he held me, all night. We didn't have sex. In the morning, he made tea for me in the little kitchenette, brought it to me in bed.

"Hey, thank you," I said.

"I love you, Erin."

The blood rushed to my head; my stomach roiled in protest. *Why did those words petrify me?* He stroked my forehead and his eyes registered the recoil I had in mine.

"You don't love me. You don't even know me."

What was it with me? It was getting to the point where whenever a man was actually nice to me, actually showed that he cared, I felt angry. I was convinced that it was a trick, a sham— or that they were only in love with some fake Erin. I was so scared that when they saw the real one, they'd laugh and take back everything they said. It was so much easier to only allow the concept of love in when it felt far away, when it felt impossible. The second it was right in front of me, I felt compelled to push it away and look for it somewhere else. It was a lie that I didn't want it; I *wanted* to be loved. But losing it was so much more painful than running away from it, or so I'd convinced myself. My reaction to love had become a compulsion. The intoxication of withholding was too strong. I wanted, I needed that control.

"I think I should go," I said.

He was visibly stunned and hurt. I felt myself go into this autopilot protection mode. I wanted to say, *No, I'm sorry, I'll stay.* But the words were locked inside me.

He grabbed his leather jacket off the floor and left me alone in the room. My body burned with what I'd just done, what I pushed away. I sat there for a moment and gritted my teeth to prevent myself from crying. I dug my nails into my wrists and counted while holding my breath. I got dressed and left, too.

By my twenty-first birthday, in November of 1994, I'd moved again, into a two-bedroom apartment just off Los Feliz Boulevard. Brett and I were idling along in an open relationship and Keith was still in and out of my life.

I was packing for Las Vegas. My dad was taking me and a few friends there to celebrate my twenty-first birthday. The phone rang; it was Keith. He called to wish me a happy birthday and wanted to take me away for the weekend.

"I'm actually going to Las Vegas. My dad planned a little thing for my birthday," I said.

"Oh. Can I come? Or can I meet up with you there?"

"Well, I mean, other people are going, too..."

"Fuck, Erin. Are you seriously still stringing that guy along?"

"I'm not stringing him along. And yes, my boyfriend is coming on the trip."

I heard what sounded like the phone being slammed against something.

"Keith..."

"No, you know what? This is bullshit. What the fuck am I doing? You've ruined my life. Do you hear me? You have ruined my fucking life, and I let you. Have a nice fucking birthday."

He hung up on me. When he did, I believed we would speak again, believed that he would still be in my life. But I never saw him again. It's shocking that we have never run into each other over the years. I have always felt badly about how I treated Keith. He wasn't perfect, but he showed up for me whenever I asked him to, and he desperately wanted to love me. I wanted him to; I wanted to love him back. I just couldn't.

In February of 1995, I got another phone call. It was a rainy night. I was home with my roommate Chris, watching an episode of *Beverly Hills, 90210* that we had recorded onto VHS. The phone rang. It was Polly. I could hardly understand what she was saying; she was sobbing on the phone. Then I finally understood what she was saying—it was Ian. Ian had died.

My knees buckled. I dropped the phone and fell to the floor. Chris took the phone, speaking quietly to Polly in the hallway. I felt both hollow and flat. Even though it had been a couple of years since I'd seen Ian, I'd naively thought that somehow, someday, we would find our way back to each other. I had clung to this belief, even though he'd gotten married and I knew he was sick.

That night, Chris convinced me to go out, to get my mind off things. Fueled by Vicodin and vodka, we met Polly at Lava Lounge, a bar on La Brea in a little strip mall. I was a regular there. Because of my haircut and the overwhelming popularity of *Pulp Fiction*, the bartenders called me "Mia Wallace." We walked in, and my favorite bartender switched the music up to "Girl, You'll Be a Woman Soon." It was a thing he did whenever I was there. I smiled; I went through the motions of talking and drinking and trying to pretend that the love of my young life hadn't just died. I looked around the bar at all the familiar faces. They didn't bring me comfort. They made me want to run. I shut my eyes and imagined myself walking out the door and right into traffic, or hitching a ride and letting myself be taken anywhere else, somewhere I could start a new life, and let go of every part of this one.

CHAPTER 8
Je T'aime... Moi Non Plus
Paris, May 1995

I rested my forehead against the cold window and looked up at the clouds moving in the gray sky like wisps of smoke. As the train descended into the Gare du Nord among the mansard rooftops, the domes of Sacré-Cœur in the distance, I knew in my body that this city and I were destined for each other. I stopped breathing for a minute and took it in. I'd gone on the trip to Europe with a friend from work. She was going to a tattoo convention in Amsterdam and I—still mourning Ian's death—wanted to go and see and escape. Our original travel plans changed, and we ended up spending the second half of the trip in Paris, where we would stay with a friend of hers. I'd never had a strong desire to visit Paris, but that all changed when our night train from Amsterdam arrived there on a cool morning in May.

I spent ten days there—buying fresh strawberries at the green market, visiting the famous cemetery Père Lachaise, sitting on the steps of the Opéra Bastille, flirting with guys and practicing my paltry French, eating fresh baguette while we strolled through neighborhoods with no agenda other than to explore, wandering the darkened rooms filled with pastels in the Musée d'Orsay, sitting in awe on the top floor of Sainte-Chapelle, taking in all the colors in stained glass.

When I got home, I began planning my move. Chris decided he wanted to move, too. It was going to be perfect. We'd sublet our apartment and go on this adventure together. My parents were supportive of this move. I was going to go back to school. I enrolled in a program at the Sorbonne for international students and began practicing my high school French. My pill pilfering stopped, too.

Lila and I spent a lot of time together in the months leading up to my move—she was living in San Francisco and I was moving to Paris but we talked incessantly and made trips up and down the coast of California to see each other. She was the one person I felt I could confide in the most about the feelings I struggled with. We talked about my dreams about Ian and how I could still feel his energy, even smell him. She understood. We promised to write to each other weekly. I wasn't bringing my heavy desktop computer with me and would have limited email access. And in the era before smartphones, my cell phone wasn't going to work in Europe. On the eve of my departure, I sat down with Brett with the intention of breaking up with him, but we left things vague—I knew it was a mistake. I should have just let him go.

My dad flew with me and my six suitcases to Paris to help me secure an apartment. I found a lovely three-room flat in a quiet neighborhood in the fifteenth arrondissement. Chris arrived a couple of weeks later, and we started setting up our life in Paris. Lila and I did write long letters to each other; we even recorded cassette tape letters à la *Felicity*. We kept our letters and tapes all of these years. When I look at them now, I have a near day-by-day chronicle of my time in Paris. They are equal parts bittersweet, cringe-worthy, and endearing.

21/09/95 Chris and I had so much fun last night. We went barhopping in the Marais. We ran into our friends Olivier and Stefan. We got plastered and they took us to this gay bar, Banana Café, over in Les Halles at 3 a.m. It was fun but so crowded and sweaty. As we walked along the river, on our way home, I felt so alive and so fucking happy to be here. It's now Monday night. I feel a little bit down right now b/c we were listening to the radio, station hopping, and "Nothing Compares 2 U" was on and I was telling Chris how it reminded me of Ian b/c it was so popular when we broke up. Then, all of a sudden, it hit me. I realized he is dead. It really freaked me out. How could I have forgotten for a moment that I'll never have the chance (in this life) to see him.

I was intoxicated by the city. I kept thinking I saw Ian—on side streets, in the corners of dark bars. I questioned if I'd ever love someone again, the way I loved him. Chris struggled to find his footing in Paris and at the end of October wanted to move back to LA.

Luckily, I'd met Faith. Faith and I were enrolled in the same program at the Sorbonne. She was in Paris for the year from Chicago, wanting to improve her French as a postgrad. We became friends effortlessly, both Scorpios, born on the same day—November 20. She looked a lot like Jennifer Aniston on *Friends*. When we went out, I got called "Mia Wallace," and she got called "Rachel." She was in a terrible living situation, and it worked out perfectly that when Chris moved out, she moved in.

We had a host of visitors. My mom came for two weeks. She arrived a bit shaken. She'd just ended things with Dave, after years of being off and on, and she'd had to put our beloved dog, Kasey, to sleep. She was devastated. Kasey had been a constant companion for her, through all her relationships and me moving out. That trip with Mom visiting is one of my fondest memories.

We had a blast. Every day she would come to meet up with Faith and me at the Jardin du Luxembourg near school. The park was resplendent in gold and red and orange leaves. Fall in Paris is glorious. We went to museums, took a couple of day trips, took in the golden city of lights at night, in the crisp air, and ran around Paris like sisters.

In November, Lila came to visit. On November 20, Faith's and my birthday, we all went to the Sans Sanz, a two-story bar in the Bastille. We sat at a corner table upstairs and met three French guys who were attractive and funny and spoke broken English. We gave them the phone number to our apartment, and I didn't think any more about it.

I went home for the holiday break in December and continued to keep things undefined with Brett. When I returned to Paris in January, the city was gray and cold, the kind of cold that gets into your bones. I felt depressed and homesick. Then Vincent called.

Vincent was one of the French guys Faith and I had met on our birthday in November. We had run into him and his friends a couple of times since we'd first met, and I found myself more and more attracted to him. He was fit and fairly tall, with dark brown hair and eyes that look at you sideways, studying you, and large soft lips. The chemistry between us was palpable. He had that same simmering sexual energy as Keith, the kind that you feel in the room and makes you turn around.

He'd called that Saturday to invite us to a party. After a long night out that involved multiple parties, we all ended up back at our apartment. Vincent and I stayed up all night talking. As he spoke, all I could focus on were those very full lips. But he held back and waited to kiss me in the morning, just before they left. I couldn't figure him out and it only made me want him more.

The next day, he called and asked if he could see me. I felt anxious all day; he'd sounded odd on the phone. I chain-smoked and watched French music videos and picked at my cuticles.

It was a quiet and frigid Sunday night. We sat in the dimly lit den in my apartment. His body language was stiff. The wide floorboards creaked as he shifted in his chair.

"I had such a good time with you last night. You know, talking to you, and I feel a strange connection."

I nodded. I felt it, too.

"But I haven't been honest with you."

I waited for him to finish his sentence. "Okay..."

"I have a girlfriend. Joan. We've been with each other for five years, since high school. And I love her very much."

"So, why did you kiss me? Why didn't you tell me this last night when we talked about everything else?" I asked.

"I don't know."

I exhaled and looked at the antique wooden desk in the corner, trying to figure out what to say.

"What are you thinking?" he asked.

"I don't know. What are you thinking?"

"I want us to be friends. I want you in my life. I feel sure that you're supposed to be in my life."

"Friends. Okay, I guess we'll be friends," I said. I felt disappointed, crushed.

He stood up, so I did, too.

"I have to go," he said, reaching his arms out to hug me.

I looked over his shoulder, out through the frosty window. Across the street, a small light illuminated the profile of a woman reading by the window. I felt a rush of sadness. Vincent pulled back and looked at me, took my face in his hands like he could feel what was happening inside me. Our hearts beat against each other through our wool sweaters. He stroked my cheek and kissed me softly on the forehead, then on the mouth. We stood there kissing for what might have been thirty minutes or thirty seconds. He pulled away and said, "I'm sorry, Erin. I have to go."

He left, and I went into Faith's room and flopped down on her bed, telling her what happened. We stayed up late, curled up together on the small daybed in the den, watching badly dubbed French reruns of *Beverly Hills, 90210*. After Faith went to bed, I recorded a long-winded tape for Lila, detailing every moment that had transpired over the weekend. By the time I was done, it was early morning, but the winter sky remained opaque. I lay down in my bed and stared at the ceiling and thought about Vincent's kisses and the way he smelled and I didn't get one bit of sleep.

The next week, Faith and I went out for a drink, back at the Sans Sanz, where we'd met Vincent. He was there with the guys, and his girlfriend, Joan. He was stiff and didn't smile when we said hello, giving me the perfunctory French greeting—a kiss on each cheek. Joan straightened her back when he introduced us and I knew she knew, the way women know. She was petite and gorgeous, mixed race with an afro and flawless skin. I felt so ugly in front of her. I could feel the world spinning beneath me and I didn't know how to stay upright. My tapes and letters for Lila were what kept me from losing my mind in the days that followed.

Hi, it's now Mon. afternoon 22/01/96. I just got back from my oral exam. Oh God, Lila, I don't want to get hurt and I don't want anyone else to get hurt, including his girlfriend. I'm feeling only about a billion emotions @ the moment. I'm going to take a long hot bath. Hopefully that will calm my nerves. I still can't fucking eat. This morning I forced myself to eat 2 tangerines. I got your letter today. Thank you. :-) Your letters always brighten my day. I love you and miss you so much. You really helped me a lot on the phone last night. No one understands me like you do…

Vincent and I continued spending time together "as friends" which invariably turned into heavy make-out sessions that crept further and further toward sex. I called Brett and ended things, finally. I even told him about Vincent. We had devolved enough from lovers to friends that this ending wasn't dramatic.

"He's never going to leave his girlfriend," he said. I feared he was right. I was frustrated and sad. Somehow this boy-man had reopened my heart and, worse still, I couldn't have him, not all of him. The role reversal of the past few years was painful. I wondered if this was my karma.

13/02/96 Hi, I'm home now, in between classes. What is wrong with me? I haven't felt this way in so long. I'm petrified. I have absolutely no control over my emotions. I fucking hate this. Valentine's Day is tomorrow. Blech!! I fucking hate it. I hate love. Remember how I told you in the last tape that I've been thinking a lot about Ian and I dreamed about him? Well, the other day I was here by myself and was sort of talking to him (in my head) and I heard his voice, not in my head but in the apt. He said, "Erin." I jumped and was so freaked. I started fully crying. :-(I was asking him to help me b/c I'm afraid of what I'm feeling. Lila, someone needs to help me seriously. My feelings for Vincent are overwhelming and I don't know if it's him or me. I feel like I can't breathe.

15/02/96 I'm home, in between classes. Lila, I can't stop bawling. I feel like someone has taken my heart out of its cage and now it's just dangling there. Is this my karma for breaking other's hearts? I feel like God has said, "Okay, you can fall in love but only to torture yourself." Maybe it's a gift. If nothing else, I've learned in Paris that I can love.

Vincent and I had a snowball fight on the banks of the Seine, in front of the Place de la Concorde, on a magical February night. The streetlights made the snow golden, and we slid down gilded patches of ice into each other's arms and made confessions and grand declarations, as kids passing by doused us with powder, because it was Mardi Gras.

Back at my apartment, we lay in bed under a heap of duvet, naked. It was far too cold to go outside, and we were starving. Starved from hours, maybe days, of learning the contours of our intertwined bodies. I remember there being chestnut cream and crème fraîche in a big white ceramic bowl, swirled together, and a sprig of mint, and spoon-feeding, and bliss.

A few weeks later, we sat in his parents' living room in a suburb of France as he recovered from an emergency appendectomy and felt electricity shoot through our fingertips and into each other. We hallucinated on infatuation and lust and passion and falling in love. But there was Joan. And every time he left me, he left with admonitions of what we'd done, of who he'd become. I was his bliss and his shame.

Some days, that shame would embed itself deep inside me. I'd wander the city and go to the Cathédrale Notre-Dame and sit on one of the long, narrow pews in the dim light and close my eyes and cry and wonder if Vincent was with Joan, naked under a heap of duvet, telling her he loved her. I prayed to a god I didn't understand, didn't know if I believed in, to give me the strength to extricate myself from him.

Other days, I'd go to the Musée d'Orsay and stand in front of my favorite painting, *Le Lit*, painted by Henri de Toulouse-Lautrec in 1892. The oil painting shows a couple, two little brunette heads, in bed, covers up to their chins, tousled hair. I had a postcard of the painting taped on the wall next to my bed. There is something about the intimacy—the emotional intimacy—in the painting that has always struck me. It's what I longed for and pushed away all at once. Maybe I only pursued it from Vincent because I couldn't really have it, not when Joan was forever in the background.

Meanwhile, Faith had her own crisis brewing. She had a boyfriend back home, whom she missed. She left Paris suddenly, after a drunken night she regretted. I was devastated when she left. I was all alone in that apartment on Avenue Félix-Faure, and I felt myself shrinking. I had no pills. Instead, I had cigarettes and long sleepless nights recording cassettes and writing letters to Lila. Occasionally, I'd break down and call her, easily spending $100 just to hear her voice.

A short while after Faith left Paris, Katie moved in. Katie was another American I met in the program at the Sorbonne. She was a strong, classic all-American blonde from Vermont, and much as it had been with Faith, our friendship quickly clicked into place. But our friendship was not quite enough to keep me from unraveling.

While Vincent and I blurred the lines between friendship and having an affair, I fooled around with other men; without any drugs, I needed sex to distract me from what I was feeling, to give me some feeling of control. They were: the young, rich American heir to a publishing empire, on permanent holiday in Paris and who lived on cocaine and candy; an old French friend I knew from LA who was visiting his dad in Paris; the American executive who would take Faith and me out to dinner when we had no money to eat and always paid for drinks and cabs; the French-Vietnamese painter with a heroin problem; the Swedish scientist. But none of them were Vincent. He knew little about my dalliances and what he did know drove him mad. So, I lied to him, as if he were my boyfriend, as I'd done in so many other relationships.

Vincent and I continued our affair well into the summer. As the lease for my apartment was coming up, I had a decision to make. I could stay another year in Paris or go back to Los Angeles, back to school at USC.

"I want you to go back to LA," he said one night in bed.

"You do?"

"Yes. And I want to go with you. I'm going to end things with Joan."

"Are you sure?"

"I'm sure. I don't want to lose you. I don't want to lose what we have. I want to make a new life with you. I want to get out of Paris and be with you."

And with that, we made plans to return to Los Angeles together. I was terrified.

CHAPTER 9
Dirty Blue Balloons
November 1996

I had waited for the man I loved to make up his mind. He did. Vincent chose me, and we left Paris and moved to Los Angeles, where he immediately began doubting his decision. He should have told me, but he didn't. I sensed it, and the doubt worked like a knife, whittling me down.

Vincent and I lived with my mom when we first got back to Los Angeles, the plan being to save money and figure out our next steps. Before Vincent arrived, my mom and I had peeled off that old Laura Ashley wallpaper and redid my room. I also got a puppy—a Rhodesian ridgeback I named Gideon. I was back in school at USC and working as a freelance wardrobe stylist, mostly for commercials. If you saw Burger King or Jack in the Box or Folgers or Sprite or Power 106 commercials in the late 1990s, there's a good chance I worked on them.

The two and a half months Vincent and I lived together were awful. They were having everything you thought you wanted only to realize you had nothing at all. Vincent was distant and sad. When we had sex, I had the same feeling I'd had with him in Paris—I was his bliss and his shame.

By late September, I'd started using crystal meth and pills again. In October, I found a letter he wrote to Joan, left carelessly in the trunk of my Jetta, telling her he loved her and wanted her back and that he'd made a huge mistake. In turn, I didn't come home that night, staying out late with a surfer guy from one of my film classes who talked like Jeff Spicoli, and had bad sex on his denim couch. When I returned the next morning, I lied about where I'd been and told Vincent he should leave. Every part of my body hurt.

By early November, he was living with his cousin in Hollywood and making plans to return to France. I stopped eating. I wanted to disappear. I wanted the thick, sucking hole of depression to vacuum me up. I spent time with Polly and Milo. I frequently drove up to San Francisco to visit Lila, usually in the middle of the night, running on crystal meth and sadness, where we'd spend weekends high on crystal, going to clubs, talking, reading tarot cards, and writing term papers.

I also rekindled a friendship with my friend Amy, who I'd worked with at the boutique. Amy was a few years older than me—Filipino by way of Texas, smart, and beautiful. Her face always struck me as the kind you'd find in a Renaissance painting, with a question behind the slight smile, something that made you want to get closer.

On my twenty-third birthday, Amy and her boyfriend, Jay, took me out to a dive bar near Jay's place in Venice, and introduced me to their friend Riley. Riley was a babe with a boyish face, deviant smile, and bright eyes—all-American and a total opposite to Vincent in every way. We spent the night together and started dating casually.

The other thing happening around me, casually, was heroin. Amy and Jay had been smoking it. I'd promised myself I wouldn't do it again. I stuck to pills and crystal meth and not eating and men, which I rationalized as healthier options.

I spent New Year's Eve in Las Vegas with Amy, Jay, Riley, and other friends. By midnight, I was drunk, and we were back in our suite, everyone there to re-up on their drug of choice. I checked my cell phone. I had messages, several of them, all from Vincent. He was drunk, too. At least, I think he was drunk. It was morning, New Year's Day in Paris.

"You're just going on with your life? You just don't give a fuck about me anymore?" he yelled at me when I called him back.

"You did this. You did this to us. Fuck you," I said and hung up the phone.

I was furious. Amy and Jay were smoking heroin in the other bedroom. I stood in the doorway between the two rooms and some small door in my brain opened, a door that had been closed since I was a teenager. *It wouldn't be so bad if I smoked a little.* I walked over to Amy and asked her if I could have some. She handed me a square piece of tinfoil with a small brown piece of tar heroin on it, a lighter, and a foil straw.

I held the tinfoil in my left hand, trembling, not because I was nervous about doing heroin again for the first time in more than eight years, but because I was so damn angry at Vincent, at myself. I put the straw in my mouth, flicked the lighter on with my right hand, and heated up the foil, inhaling the sick, sweet, smoke. It tasted different than I remembered, maybe because I'd never smoked it like this. I'd only shot it or snorted it. *This isn't so bad*, I thought. *At least I'm not using a needle.*

The heroin brought me a familiar, swift, and total reprieve from the anger, anxiety, and sadness I'd felt only moments before. *Yes. Yes. This is what I need.*

Heroin was officially back in my life. I was using on weekends, and then on weekends and Wednesdays, and then every damn day. I managed to keep up with school, take hikes in Runyon Canyon with Gideon, and still take freelance styling jobs. *How could this be bad? I'm doing so well.*

I moved out of my mom's, back again to Beachwood Canyon. This time to Monroe Manor, an iconic, terraced mid-century building known for being Joey Tribiani's building in the *Friends* spinoff, *Joey*, and supposedly named after Marilyn Monroe. I loved that apartment. It was a one-bedroom with hardwood floors, original green tiles in the bathroom, a small office, and a large private patio, walled in with ivy. My first night there, I made myself a bed on the living room floor, put on a vintage slip—which was my lounging outfit of choice in those days— curled up next to Gideon, smoked heroin and Winston Lights, ate peanut M&M's, and watched a VHS tape of *Kalifornia* while nodding out. This was heaven. There were few things I enjoyed more in 1997 than nodding out in a slip while eating peanut M&M's and smoking, snuggled with Gideon.

As smoothly as things seemed to be moving along, I had an annoying voice in my head that I couldn't shake, the one that said, *You might just be strung out, little girl.* I couldn't remember the last day I went without getting high. I wondered if I'd feel sick if I skipped a day. But each time that nagging voice got loud, I smoked more dope and pushed it aside. *I'm fine. I'm doing great. Haven't been happier in a long time.*

I'd sometimes buy from Amy and Jay's friend and bandmate. She was a small-time dealer, really just did it to support her own habit. She'd lower the drugs in a small bucket out her window, New York City–style. A few times, I'd buy from this older witchy woman who dealt out of an occult shop in Atwater Village. They were both unreliable. When all else failed, I'd head to Sixth and Bonnie Brae for a drive-through.

The corner of Sixth Street and Bonnie Brae sits in the West- lake district, just northeast of MacArthur Park, near Alvarado Street, a stone's throw from downtown LA. I usually had Gideon with me, a silent witness in my passenger seat, sitting there noble and only a little accusingly with his nose in the air. In 1997, you could drive up to the northeast corner, in front of the doughnut shop, and buy drugs. Window down, a Mexican or Guatemalan man would break off from the small group standing in the parking lot and approach. "Four cheeba," I'd say, holding up four fingers. Within seconds, he'd scoop the inside of his cheek and slide four blue balloons into my hand, as I slid $80 into his. I'd shove the balloons into my pocket and drive away. The quality was usually consistent on that corner. It was managed by MS-13. But if the corner was cold, and the cops were out, I'd have to look elsewhere.

Looking elsewhere led to me roaming MacArthur Park at 2:00 a.m. in my favorite getting-high outfit—a vintage slip and flip-flops—dope-sick and sweaty. Looking elsewhere led to me buying shit dope off some rando on Burlington that was barely strong enough to get me well. And looking elsewhere led to a stranger I let into my car on Alvarado who gave me crack shavings instead of heroin. I hit him and screamed and he was so put off by my erratic behavior that he threw my money back at me, grabbed his crack, and spit on my car as I drove away, muttering in Spanish. The only thing I caught was *puta loca*. I shook, my hands gripping the wheel. I was strung out. There was no denying it. I didn't know what scared me more—that I was using a couple hundred dollars a day of dope or that I didn't know if I cared.

Vincent sent me letters, many letters, telling me how he missed me, loved me, how sorry he was. All I could think of when I looked at those letters was the other letter I'd found in the trunk of my car—the letter to Joan, the one saying all the same things to her he was now saying to me. *I don't believe a fucking word.*

One day early that spring, at USC, I was walking down the hall from the French department and saw a petite olive-skinned brunette with striking blue eyes who resembled the actress Claire

Forlani. I knew who it was instantly. It was Diana, an old friend of mine. Diana and Polly had a falling-out a couple of years prior and we had drifted apart as a result. Diana and I chatted for over an hour, like no time had passed, standing in that hallway. That night she came over and I smoked heroin in front of her. I had to; at that point, I couldn't go for more than a few hours without a fix. It was either kick her out or let her in on my secret. Other than Amy and Jay, I'd been hiding my using from everyone. She was nonjudgmental and we hung out as if I were not nodding out mid-conversation on my vintage couch.

Diana started going with me when I scored, and brought me peanut M&M's and watched movies with me. She was escaping her own problems with her inattentive live-in boyfriend, who was like a ghost, existing in time and space with her, but not in spirit. Looking back, I think she needed someone to take care of, to focus on. Finally, eventually, curiosity got the best of her and she tried heroin for the first time. And she didn't stop. We didn't stop. I covered the pangs of guilt I felt over dragging her into my addiction by getting higher, getting to that heroin low.

One afternoon, I found myself driving to Jay's apartment in Venice with Polly. Amy and Jay had left some heroin for me. I hadn't intended for her to be in the car with me, but she was fighting with Milo. I felt dope-sick and would need to get high before we drove back to Hollywood. Heroin was in the air in 1997; I felt emboldened by the casualness with which others were using. *Fuck it*, I thought.

"So, Polly, I kind of need to tell you something before we get there."

"Yeah?"

"I've kind of been dabbling with heroin on occasion—I mean, I'm not strung out and no needles."

She looked stunned, shook her head, and let out a half laugh.

"Do you think I'm a total loser?" I asked.

"Erin. I need to tell *you* something."

"What?"

"Well, the reason that Milo and I are fighting is we've been trying to kick. We've been 'dabbling,' too," she said, making air quotes with her hands. "And we *are* just a little strung out."

"Shit, I'm sorry. I won't do any in front of you."

"Erin," she said, widening her eyes.

Relief came to the surface of my skin. I knew it was on. I knew we were going to get high together. I knew that I was about to go lower. And I wasn't going alone. That night, back in Polly's apartment at the bottom of Nichols Canyon, I shot up. There was no more denying being strung out or my no-needle rule.

The drugs brought Polly and Diana back together. Diana started shooting up, too, although she was markedly less strung out than the rest of us. This was uncharted territory for me. My drug use had always been solo; now I had a whole peer group that was using to varying degrees. Through Milo and Polly, I got a new dealer—Juan. His dope was good, he was reliable, and I didn't have to drive to Sixth and Bonnie Brae anymore.

Once or twice a week, I'd drive over to a pop-up table on the sidewalk of a quiet side street just off of La Brea, set up by Clean Needles Now, to get new needles, alcohol swabs, tiny sterile cotton balls, and latex tourniquets. I'd bring my needles back, the sharps and bodies separated into two large ziplock bags. I will always be grateful for Clean Needles Now and other programs that replaced them. They are *the* reason I don't have HIV or Hepatitis C, and I know they saved thousands of lives besides my own.

Lila moved back from San Francisco, and while she wasn't using heroin, she was using crystal meth. I'd go to her new apartment and stay up on crystal, talking all night, eating small bites of Kahlúa cream cheese pie from Marie Callender's. This didn't last long. Lila was preparing to go to law school and she had to stop using. She made the decision and did it. *I can do that,*

I thought. *I will do that. I'll give myself two more weeks.* But I didn't or couldn't. After she decided to quit, we hung out much, much less, and I lied to her about how much and how often I was using.

In between all the scoring and getting high, I continued dating. I was still dating Riley, off and on. I dated a musician who lied about having a girlfriend and thought I had an eating disorder, which sounded better to me than an addiction so I didn't deny it. I dated a VP at Paramount Studios who'd gone to Harvard, drove a Saab, always wore a sports coat, liked to eat at The Ivy, and enjoyed smoking crack on the weekends. I dated another friend of Amy and Jay, who I slept with and panicked when he told me he had feelings for me, jumping out of a second-story window into the boxwood hedges below. But none of them filled the hole left by Vincent.

Diana graduated from USC that May. By graduation, we were spending almost every day together—watching movies and old reruns of *Beverly Hills, 90210* in her bed while her boyfriend was at work. She had a graduation trip coming up. She was going to Europe and would be spending a few days in Paris. I emailed Vincent, asking if he could meet up with her when she was there, so she'd know someone in the city. Because no one checked their email with any frequency back then, it took him some time to answer. He wrote back: "Of course."

One night while Diana was in Paris, she called me. It was late there. She'd spent the evening with Vincent and his friends, and they spent most of that time talking about me. She told me that he loved me, that he was still in love with me, that she believed him, that maybe I should give him another chance. I got off the phone with her and turned on the TV and lit a cigarette. *Is he the one? I do love him. I've never stopped loving him.*

The next day, Vincent called. We talked for a long time about what had happened and where we were now. He told me about everything that had gone on since he went back to Paris. He'd briefly dated Joan again, before finally ending it, had been focusing on figuring out what he wanted to do with his life. He hadn't been dating anyone else and he was assuredly, wholly in love with me.

"I love you, too," I said. "There's no one else for me either."

I was such a liar. I'm not talking about the men I'd conveniently omitted from the conversation, but heroin. Heroin was what *was* for me. Heroin was the thing that separated me from him, from everyone else. And I didn't say one word about it.

In June, I went back to France to spend six weeks with Vincent. I got on that plane with a layer of naivete and denial so thick I couldn't see straight. I arrived in Paris sick. It was the flu, I told him. I was miserable. I'd never been that dope-sick before. After the worst part of withdrawal was over, the guilt stuck to me, immobilizing my thoughts. We were in bed, watching *Pulp Fiction* of all things, and I had to say *something*.

"Vincent, I need to tell you something."

"Did you fuck someone?"

"What?"

"You fucked someone else in LA?" he asked, his voice shaking.

"No." *Liar. Liar.*

"You know how when I was a teenager, I experimented with drugs a little bit… Well, I sort of did the same thing again. I was just so sad and—"

"What did you take?"

Am I going to really tell him the truth?

"What did you take?"

"I mean, pills mostly. But a couple times, I smoked heroin."

"Heroin? You took heroin? Are you fucking kidding me? Did you use a needle?"

"No." *Liar. Liar. Liar.*

When Vincent and I argued, or had any sort of heated conversation, we did so bilingually. Back and forth, he spoke French and I answered in English. Thinking how silly we must have sounded, I laughed.

"You think it's funny? You think this is a joke?" he asked.

"No. And I'm sorry."

Vincent believed that the problem was Los Angeles. He took me away to the countryside, to his grandparents' home in the mountains of Auvergne. It was healing and magical.

I spent my mornings with his grandmother, at the old farmhouse table in their kitchen. We'd drink coffee, and I'd have small slices of baguette with fresh butter out of a crock and sometimes homemade cherry preserves.

We spent our days walking through their small village, and the people would wave and say, "Hello, American." We went to the mineral baths and took long walks and stopped to talk to the cows. I took photographs on film that I would never develop and we visited the Laguiole knife workshop.

In the evenings, we'd sit by candlelight, and his grandfather, stroking the head of his ancient wobbly black dog, would tell us stories about the town and the French resistance fighters.

Auvergne gave me hope. I started to feel human again without drugs in my system.

When we returned to Paris, Vincent asked me to marry him and I said yes. We made a plan. He would come back to LA in September and we would get married the following year and then return to France after I'd finished school.

The day before I left, we went to the Clingnancourt flea market, the Marché aux Puces de Saint-Ouen, on the northwestern edge of the city. We found a small antique diamond ring that he bought for me, and he knelt down, right there, among the rows and rows of antique stalls, and put the ring on my finger. *You can do this. You can be happy. You can stay clean.*

Diana picked me up from LAX in her little black Mazda.

"How was it? Show me the ring!" she said when I got in the car.

I showed her my left hand.

"Aw, it's so pretty. How do you feel?"

I waited for a moment to answer because I didn't know how I felt. We pulled up to a stoplight on Century Boulevard.

"Well, I know I've got six weeks left before I have to stop getting high."

She looked at me.

"Do you have any?" I asked.

She raised her eyebrows. I couldn't wait to get home. We pulled off on a side street and I shot up in the passenger seat. After throwing up on the sidewalk, I got back in the car, put my sunglasses on, put the seat back, lit a cigarette, and said, "Okay, let's go. I'm good."

CHAPTER 10
The Green Sweater
New York City, August 1997

It was 5:00 a.m., and I was wide-awake—the kind of awake with edges so sharp that sleep is carved away. Chills marched on my skin like an army of ants, and I searched in the dark for my green sweater. I had been wearing that sweater incessantly since I'd returned from Paris. The sweater went on and then was pulled off, repeatedly, each day, in my desperate, yet half-hearted, attempts at kicking. It was pale green, woven of silk and cashmere, bought in one of the shopping sprees I went on to distract myself from the hundreds of dollars a day I was shooting in my arm, and it filled me with comfort and disgust in equal measure. It wasn't even a great color on me; it wasn't really me. Maybe that's why I bought it. Hiding had become my occupation.

It was August in New York. There may be no worse time and place to kick than August in New York. Heat and humidity and intense smells amplify withdrawal symptoms. Everyone has their AC on full blast; you're continually flipping between hot and cold. The changes in temperature, outside and in, grated on me, irritating my prickly skin. And so, the green sweater went on and off, on and off.

I'd come back East to visit my dad, and also to try to coax myself into kicking. It was a bad idea. *Why did I always think that kicking dope on vacation would work?* My dad had moved to Rhode Island but was in New York on business, and I'd gone with him to the city. I'd done the last of my dope around nine, the night before, in my hotel bathroom. My kick was just beginning. I hated myself. I hated myself for being a junkie, for acting out that painful charade, but mostly, for not bringing more dope with me.

At 8:00 a.m., I checked the adjoining room; Dad had left for the day. I yanked the green sweater off. The fabric stuck to my damp brow as I struggled to get it over my head. I was drenched in sweat. Stumbling to the bathroom, my stomach cramped and feeling nauseous, I knew I was going to be sick. Out it came, vomit and shame and sadness and despair and more vomit. Lying down on the bathroom floor felt good, or at least better. The blue ceramic tiles soothed my clammy, achy body and let me rest, at least for a minute. I lay there and thought about how many hours of my life I'd spent on bathroom floors, studying the grout. At least this was a nice one.

Once I caught my breath, I managed to heave myself into the shower. The water played torture games on my skin. Collapsing after the shower, I lay on the bed for a few hours trying to will myself to sleep. When that didn't work, I had to get out of there.

Distractions, I needed distractions. Popping a couple of Valium, I slipped on some jeans and a tank top, and my cream-and-red Prada platforms with red leather leaves and flowers all along the sides. I still managed to look pulled together somehow, as long as you didn't look too closely. I threw the green sweater into my bag. The sweater had become like a sick security blanket.

The sunlight outside was blinding. Opiate withdrawal makes any kind of sensation too much—too bright, too loud, too scratchy. I hailed a cab and climbed in, crumpling onto the smooth back seat, and instructed the driver to head uptown, to Bergdorf Goodman, where I could pretend that I was not a twenty-three-year-old junkie in a green sweater kicking dope. The AC was on in the cab, and I was soon shivering—the sweater went back on. I was carsick and tried to take my focus off the cars and the buildings and the swarms of humans we passed. I tried to find a horizon, and when I couldn't, I shut my eyes. That fifteen-minute ride felt hours long. I overtipped the driver, handing him damp wadded cash, and flung myself out of the cab, in front of The Paris Theatre.

The city seized me—the steam and the concrete and the beat and the weight of it all. The sweater came back off. Everything was too bright, too much: the people, the noise. It was all moving too quickly, with too much determination. I stopped at a hot dog vendor for a bottle of water and gulped down half the bottle before throwing it in my purse, and I braced myself to enter the store.

The brass door felt heavier than I remembered. Cold air licked my forehead, and I was engulfed in a tornado of smells—perfume, carpet, leather, fashion, and money. The combination made me feel sicker. I headed to the bathroom to regroup. Splashing cold water on my face, I caught my eyes in the mirror and shuddered. I hated seeing my reflection—green and hollow and sick. Thinking about the night before, I got lost for a moment, standing there with the water running, avoiding my eyes.

I'd met a friend of mine, Jane, at Raoul's in Soho. I hadn't seen her for almost a year, and the last time was in Paris when we were both living there. We sat at the bar and laughed and smoked many cigarettes.

"Girl, you look fantastic," she said, and I knew it was code for skinny.

A rare moment of candor struck me, and I said, "I've been using heroin for the last nine months."

"Well, I mean, you know, the whole heroin chic is working for you!" she replied without missing a beat.

"But it's killing me," I said, laughing.

She laughed harder, and she drank a bottle of wine as I sipped on watered-down Coca-Cola and made many trips to the bathroom to shoot my dwindling supply of dope and take more Valium, trying to prolong the inevitable.

I realized the middle-aged blonde woman with a perfect blowout standing next to me was speaking.

"Miss, miss! You're wasting water."

"Thanks, sorry. Sorry."

She made a little sigh and left. I met my eyes again in the mirror and put on under-eye concealer. Silencing the germaphobe inside me, I put my mouth to the faucet and gulped enough water to swallow one more Valium. *I am ready to do this.*

The green sweater went back on, and I shopped. I didn't have the energy to try anything on. My father had given me money, had been giving me money for so long, and I had the vague passing thought that I was spending it like I was going to be dead soon. Money had been a stand-in for so many things—it was love and affection and control and illusion and, most of all, shame. If my dad didn't indulge me, didn't give me money and buy me things, I'd have proof that he did not love me. But the money made me feel ashamed and the shame pushed me to want to get rid of it, as quickly as it was given to me.

I brushed the thought away and continued chatting with the saleswoman, performing for her—playing the role of a twenty-three-year-old who had her shit together, who had money to burn, who was recently engaged, whose fiancé was arriving from France in mere weeks and had no idea his beloved was so sick. But the truth is, I was a child who was lying to everyone to varying degrees, a child who was burning through money that she didn't deserve.

The saleswoman was folding my purchases and placing them in tissue paper and talking. I couldn't hear her words any longer because my ears were ringing, and I continued to smile and perspire. The sweater came back off. She asked me if I'd like a glass of water and I was upset that she saw me sweating. I shoved the Amex in her hand and said, "No."

Looking down at my tank top, I saw that my nipples were erect and I had large sweat marks beneath my breasts and under my armpits. The chills came back, and I put the sweater back on, even though I was damp and wilting. I hated the saleswoman. I hated myself.

I had successfully distracted myself for a short amount of time and was a couple of hours further into my kick. The force of the heat outside left me instantaneously clammy, and I couldn't take one more step until the stupid green sweater came off again. My dad was picking me up at six. It was only four. I figured I could kill time in The Palm Court. The Palm Court sits in the Plaza Hotel, across from Bergdorf Goodman. I had been coming there for tea since I was seven.

The maître d' seated me with a beautiful view of the pianist and violin player. I loved it there. The gold and the green and the ridiculous opulence made me feel like a little girl again. I ordered my high tea. Soon there would be crumpets and clotted cream, tea sandwiches, strawberries and whipped cream, and of course, the tea. Before I could enjoy any of it, a cold sweat gripped me. Cramping muscles followed.

I looked around the room and saw the old-timers and the tourists, a family, and a mother and little girl. Everyone was seated with someone. Everyone but me. The loneliness was palpable and coated my tongue. I couldn't control the tears welling up. The people at the table next to me spoke in hushed tones and glanced at me, and I wondered if they were trying to figure out what was wrong with me. Their whispers joined forces with the piano and the violin and became a loud, dissonant symphony. My ears rang.

Off to the bathroom, I went. I clutched my purse and my sweater together like a makeshift life raft. The bathroom, down the long, carpeted hall, past the painting of Eloise, past the chocolate shop, past the gift shop, was empty. The bathroom attendant was at the door, and I couldn't look at her. I stood in front of the mirror and faced myself. *Maybe I look too thin. Shit, the last time I weighed myself, I was 110, but I think I've lost more weight since then. I'm only five-eight, and there are plenty of models who are five-ten and weigh less. But you're not a model, Erin.*

My long dark hair looked greasy, even though I'd washed it that morning and it was in a ponytail. I could see my heart beating in the vein in my neck. The bathroom attendant came up next to me and placed a towel on the counter. We made eye contact in the mirror. There was familiarity in the gaze. I looked down and turned on the water, but I didn't wash my hands. *I know her eyes.* I was pretty sure she was the same bathroom attendant who had been there for years, since I was a little kid, for as long as I could remember. I turned off the water and looked up again. She was back against the wall but still looking at me with sad eyes. The circles under her eyes were almost as dark as mine, and I wondered where hers came from. I felt like throwing up.

Sitting down on the toilet, I put my head in my hands and wept. *Fuck you.* I felt hot. The sweater came off. As I began to fold the sweater in my lap, I noticed something stuck in the rolled collar. Slowly I unrolled the collar. Boom. *How is this possible?*

It was a piece—no, a chunk—of tar heroin. Relief (and a little guilt) washed over me. I pulled a pencil case out of my bag. I kept my gear in there, organized in a pink plastic box with Hello Kitty's benign white kitty face on it. I took out the small spoon and lighter, grabbed the water bottle from my purse, and poured a little bit into the spoon with half of the heroin. I heated it and plopped the tiny cotton ball in the liquid, before drawing it up into a fresh needle. I didn't care if the woman outside knew. It was like junkie Christmas. I shot up and leaned forward with a weighty exhale against the door. I sat there, letting myself enjoy the relief of that high. I had enough to keep me from getting too sick before flying back to LA the next day. *I'll kick when I get home*, I thought. There were still a couple more weeks before Vincent arrived.

I didn't need the green sweater anymore because I was at the perfect temperature. It all felt okay. The sweater smelled of sweat and sadness. I rolled it into a ball and stuffed it inside the small trash can in the toilet stall. I walked to the sink and washed my hands in slow motion. I tipped the attendant $20 on the way out, and she watched as I passed.

CHAPTER 11
Last House at the End
of the Street
September 1997

There was a spider on the wall above the dresser next to the bathroom—the bathroom that smelled like Ajax and Betadine. I am not afraid of spiders, but I wanted to keep an eye on it. My eyes hurt and I was sure I'd never sleep again. Heroin slows everything down, dulls the edges. Now, without it, everything was sharp and amplified, and my body was revolting. Every time my hands touched my face to rub my eyes or mouth, that smell—the rotten garbage smell—made me wince. *Can other people smell it, too? I wonder if I can sneak out to the porch and have a cigarette. What time is it? 5:00 a.m.?*

It had been seven days since I'd arrived at the rehabilitation center, five days since I was released from the detox ward. It had been seven days since my whole world cracked open and swallowed everything that came before. My soul was in a constant state of wanting to claw its way right out of my skin.

Rehab so far had been a series of plastic sheets, shuffling from group to group, and the smells, the smells. My skin smelled like rancid chicken soup. For the past five days, I had been at the bungalow, white with blue trim, the last house at the end of the street, confronting the mess I made. *I am a heroin addict.*

August had been a blur of false starts, a carousel of going through withdrawal into *Oh, I'll kick tomorrow, I may as well as enjoy this while I can.* Instead of kicking heroin, I got another dog—a rescued Great Dane named Isabelle—because clearly pet ownership was a surefire way to stop those pesky dope cravings.

By Labor Day, a week before Vincent was to arrive, I was shooting up more than I ever had. Amy and Jay came over. I decided to take the dogs for a walk, so high I could barely string a sentence together. When I think about that day, I can picture myself, in that vintage green-and-white-checkered halter dress and brown platforms, walking up Beachwood Canyon Drive like I was walking through molasses, with two huge dogs.

I met a neighbor, a woman a little older than me with long curly red hair, who also had a dog, and she invited me to let the dogs play in her yard. I don't remember what we talked about, but I do remember waking up on a lawn chair in her yard at dusk—just me and my dogs. The neighbor was nowhere to be seen. I'd nodded out and burnt a hole with my cigarette in my dress. And I was too high to be mortified. When I got home, Amy was frantic. She'd been trying to find me; I'd been gone for hours. When I undressed later for my shower, I realized that I'd also thrown up a little on my dress. I wondered if I'd fallen out—overdosed.

Vincent arrived a week later. I had cooked up and rationed out needles filled with heroin and stored them in my Hello Kitty pencil case so that I'd have them ready to go in case I needed to be quick. I should have been overjoyed when I saw him at LAX. Instead, I felt dread at how I was going to keep myself together. He ran toward me, tears of joy in his eyes, and hugged me and kissed my neck. And it was like he could feel my nervousness in our embrace.

"My love, let me look at you," he said, holding my cold hands in his. I saw the joy in his eyes shift, and a worry, a fear that maybe he wasn't even aware of, showed itself.

Later that night in bed, we lay in the dark, after reacquainting ourselves with each other's bodies. His arms around me should have felt like reunion, relief, like love. Instead, they felt like a prison. I needed my next fix.

"Erin?" he whispered.

"Yeah?"

"Something is wrong. I can feel you're so far away from me."

"I'm sorry," I said. "I'm just tired. I had a long day at school and was so excited about you getting here that I'm just…tired."

Once I knew he was asleep, I sneaked into the bathroom, unlocked the pencil case, turned the shower on, and shot up on the cold bathroom floor.

We went on like this for a couple of weeks. I'd get high in my car parked in the dark, way up by the Hollywood sign, or in bathrooms or parking garages at USC. When he was away or asleep, I'd make up a batch of needles; I couldn't go more than a few hours without a fix. Diana was getting drugs for me because factoring in the time to score was getting difficult.

On Monday, September 22, two weeks after he'd arrived, I made spaghetti for dinner. We ate, and I told him I wanted to take a bath before doing dishes. I locked myself in the bathroom and sat on the toilet opposite the old porcelain tub, in my underwear and a man's white oxford shirt with a preloaded syringe in my hand. I tied off my arm and tried to get a vein. It wasn't working; I kept missing, having to withdraw the needle and try again, poking and scraping under the skin with veins that had become uncooperative.

"Erin, are you in the bath?" Vincent asked from the other side of the door.

"Yes," I said, willing him to go away.

When I finally succeeded in hitting a vein, my relief was short-lived. I didn't undo the rubber tourniquet around my arm quickly enough, and the needle flew out of my arm, across the bathroom, landing on the green tiled floor. Seconds after it did, there was pounding on the bathroom door.

"I know what you're doing. I fucking know. Oh my God, how could you do this?" Vincent yelled.

"What? What do you mean? I'm in the bath."

"You are a liar. I know, Erin. I saw you."

"I don't know what you... What are you talking about?"

"I saw your fucking needle," he said, shoving a piece of Isabelle's chew toy under the door.

Oh my God. Could he really see under the door?

I began to panic. I grabbed the syringe and my pencil case and shoved them in my office, which was on the other side of the bathroom, through another door.

"Open the fucking door, Erin."

I tried to look composed as I unlocked the door.

"I can't believe this. I can't believe you are a fucking junkie. You have lied to me all this time? Oh my God, oh my God!"

I looked down and saw that when I made a mess of my vein, I'd bled, and that blood had dripped all over that white shirt and down my bare leg. I stood there frozen in the small hallway just outside the bathroom door while Vincent paced and screamed. The dogs hid in the bedroom. Vincent called my mom and told her I was shooting heroin. I needed to get out of that apartment. I couldn't listen to him anymore. I grabbed the phone and told her I needed her help.

In a daze, I threw on jeans, and we got in my burgundy Jetta with the dogs. Vincent drove. As we headed up over Barham and turned onto Forest Lawn Drive, I shut my eyes while he continued to alternate between muttering under his breath and yelling at me. I thought back to more than a decade earlier when

Ted and I were heading the other way on this dark road, past the cemetery and the dry riverbed. I needed an exit, any exit.

I flung open the passenger side door and fumbled with my seat belt with every intention of jumping out of the car at forty-five miles per hour. Vincent grabbed my arm and slammed on the brakes, pulling over to the shoulder of the road, right in front of the entrance to the cemetery.

"Are you fucking crazy? You're crazy now?" he screamed.

I shut the door and turned away from him, resting my head on the door. My body vibrated between the high and the adrenaline of getting caught.

My mom was eerily calm when we arrived. Vincent refused to sleep in a bed with me, so I slept on the floor in the living room, spooned between the two dogs. By early morning, I was sick. I heard my mom walking back and forth in the hallway between the dining room and living room and talking on the phone in hushed tones. When I sat up and opened my eyes, she was sitting just a few feet from me in a chair, looking at me.

"Mom," I started.

"Those were your drugs, right? The ones you told me weren't yours?" she asked, referring to a few months back when I'd spent the night and she found my balloons of heroin—that I passed off as speed I'd procured for someone else at school "to get through finals."

"Yes."

"Was that heroin?"

"Yes."

"And I just gave it right back to you," she said, exhaling and shaking her head. "How long?" she asked.

"What?"

"How long have you been using heroin?"

"Just for like a few months. Six months. I don't know."

My cheeks flushed with the lie. I felt my stomach cramping and contracting. "I'll be right back."

"Where are you going?" she asked.

"The bathroom."

"Do you have drugs on you?"

"No. And I'm gonna be sick."

When I returned to the living room, Vincent sat across from my mom with his arms crossed. He wouldn't look at me.

"I'm taking you to the hospital today, in an hour. They will detox you. And from there, you'll go to a treatment program for twenty-eight days."

It was clear my mom had been educating herself on the phone.

"Okay," I said.

What other choice did I have? I couldn't bear the thought of speaking or arguing with Vincent about this. When we left for my intake, Vincent would still not look at me and wouldn't say goodbye. I hugged my dogs and changed into a white T-shirt my mom let me borrow. I threw the bloody button-down shirt in the trash.

My mom and I drove in silence to the hospital. I was already deep enough in withdrawal that I didn't, I couldn't, feel scared about what was coming next. I was too sick. I shut my eyes and tucked my arms into the T-shirt as I shivered. I remember very little about being checked in at the hospital. I answered questions as my ears rang and my body shook. It all felt like a dream, a bad one.

At the hospital, I heard a chorus of moaning people and the cold Filipino nurses who chided me for my failure as a young woman. "Why did you do this? You're a pretty young lady. You have a nice family." They clucked their tongues and raised their eyebrows, poking and prodding. I felt like a caged thing, an experiment gone wrong.

I couldn't get my dad's face out of my head. He flew in. There I was, in the detox ward, withering away in discomfort. He walked into my little hospital room filled with yellow afternoon light, looked at me, turned around, and walked right out. I could hear him in the hallway, talking to my mom. He was crying. I have never seen my dad cry. He kept repeating, "What has she done to herself? Why? Why would she do this?"

Many years before, when I was a little girl, we'd been in the emergency room at that same hospital. I got sick frequently as a kid, and I spent many hours in doctors' offices and ERs. I was really sick at the time with pneumonia. They had to give me a large, very painful shot of antibiotics in my butt. I was scared, mostly that I was going to faint—something I did frequently in medical settings. I sat there in my flannel Laura Ashley night-gown with the little pink flowers and a plastic green bowl in my lap for throwing up. For some reason, my mom wasn't there; it was just me and my dad. To distract me, he had done his best impression of that cartoon dog—the one modeled after Lenny in *Of Mice and Men*. The big dumb dog would always say to the little one, "Which way did he go, George? Which way did he go?" My dad acted it out for me with his Persian accent: "Vich vay did he go, George? Vich vay did he go?"

I wanted to go back in time; I wanted my dad to distract me with his cartoon dog voice. But that was then.

When my mom and I first arrived at the rehab bungalow, I was petrified. One of the counselors, John, did my intake. John would become my favorite counselor there. He was six-five, black, sober for thirteen years, got clean in a Salvation Army on Skid Row. His story made me feel safe, because if he could re-cover, maybe I could, too. But during the intake, he spoke with little inflection to his voice as he went over the rules.

"Mom, please don't leave me here. Please. I can do this outpa-tient. I promise. I can't do it here. Please, please, please. I won't use again, I promise," I screeched through loud heaving sobs.

John looked at my mom and said, "You need to go now, Mom."

My mom looked back at me.

"Mom, you need to leave. She's going to be okay. But she needs help. Let us help her."

My mom got up and walked out the door.

"No!" I protested like a toddler and put my head in my lap, crying, snot running all over the place.

John gave me some tissue and a cup of water. "Okay, drink some water. Let's get you to your first group."

I wiped the tears and snot until the tissue turned into little balls. I gulped down the water, stood up, and hesitantly followed John. As we walked down the hallway, he pointed to a room on the left.

"That's your room there. Your mom left you a bag."

We walked into a sterile room with gray industrial carpeting and hard blue plastic chairs. Everyone was sitting in a circle. The air-conditioning was blasting, and I was in the same white T-shirt my mom had lent me the day she drove me to the hospital. I wasn't wearing a bra and was suddenly self-conscious. I crossed my arms to cover my nipples and slunk down in a chair next to John. He had everyone go around the room and introduce themselves, identify as alcoholics or addicts, and name their drug of choice. Everyone talking became a blur. When it was my turn, my voice cracked as I said, "I'm Erin. I'm a heroin addict."

It felt shocking to say it out loud. It was the first true thing I'd said in a long time.

As that first terrifying day wore on, I began to calm down. I attended my first twelve-step meeting that night. I was resigned to where I was—maybe solely out of exhaustion. I called my mom late that night from the payphone, wearing the blue hooded sweatshirt I was grateful she'd packed for me. When she picked up the phone, her voice sounded so small and hoarse, like she'd been crying.

"Mom?"

"Hi, honey."

"Thank you."

We sat in silence for a minute, but I could hear that she was stifling tears.

"Thank you, Mom. You did the right thing."

And I meant it.

"Honey… I am glad you're there, too. I love you."

As I settled into rehab, I was treated like a human being— a broken human being, but a human being nonetheless. There were eighteen of us broken human beings there. I was the youngest person, one of three females and the only heroin addict.

I couldn't bear to stare at that spider any longer. *Maybe Andrew will be up? Maybe we can share a smoke and flirt*, I thought. Then I thought about Vincent—the disappointment in his face, the betrayal. *He will never be able to forgive me. How could he?*

I walked into the "living room." No one else was up. This is what happens when you are the only heroin addict in a rehab full of coke fiends and meth heads. They sleep ALL the time. The alcoholics sleep, too. *Will I ever sleep again?* My legs felt liquid, like they couldn't quite hold me up. I had patches on my arm that lower your blood pressure, to help with my ongoing withdrawal. They made me feel like I was going to faint all the time, yet I still couldn't sleep. I found some smuggled-in real coffee in the kitchen. The rehab was run by an Adventist hospital. It was news to me that Adventists don't do meat or caffeine. I couldn't have cared less about the meat, but right then, I needed the caffeine.

I took my cup of coffee out to the front porch. The air felt good at dawn. Typical September in Los Angeles, the heat had been unbearable. But early-morning air was the kind you could breathe. That didn't stop me from lighting my first cigarette of the day. I saw that Dwayne was up. "Hi, Dwayne."

He smiled and shuffled past the door on his way to the kitchen. Dwayne worked for the CIA for thirty years. When he retired, he started drinking, and he nearly drank himself to death. He was shrouded in secrets and lies that he wasn't supposed to tell anyone, and it was suffocating him; he was pouring vodka straight down his throat so he could forget. I understood. Sometimes Dwayne had nightmares. I'd heard him from across the hall, yelling out in the middle of the night. I wondered if anyone else could hear him or if I was the only one.

One by one, my new roommates woke up. We had to be ready for group by seven and the first group of the day was run by John. A couple of days before at my first group meeting with my parents, John explained the concept of addiction as a family disease. My parents were not too keen on this notion. All they could see was that their daughter *was not like these people.* My father wanted me to leave rehab and go back to France. Vincent wanted me to leave rehab and go back to France. My mom talked a lot about how this was affecting her. But more and more, I was sure that I was just like these people. That I was sick and that now, for the first time, I was finally getting the kind of help I needed.

Before group, I needed to take a shower. The water hurt. I hoped it would help to wash away the bad smells and my tight muscles and the guilt I felt for ending up here. I wanted to wash away what was behind and what was ahead. I pulled my weak, wet body from the shower and got dressed, putting on a white baby T-shirt and overalls and blue Converse All Stars. Getting dressed took all of my energy. I lay down on the bed and shut my eyes. I thought about the weeks and months leading up to rehab. Shooting up in my car, before school, before work. Making excuses to leave the house, to hide in the bathroom. Lying to Vincent. My exhausted brain put the moments together in the wrong order and sped them up until I couldn't keep my eyes shut any longer. This is why I couldn't sleep. *Monsters don't sleep.* There was a knock at my door.

"Erin? It's time for group," said Andrew from the hallway.

John was there, waiting for us, in the big room with the aggressively white walls and the vertical blinds and the blue chairs. The room was cold. I was always cold because of the patches. I wrapped my arms around myself, rubbing my arms, and drew my knees up, curling into the chair awkwardly. I noticed Andrew smiling at me from a few seats away. I found him so sexy. He was ten years older than me—a dark-haired, handsome restaurateur with long eyelashes, crooked dimples, and a penchant for vodka and cocaine. *What's wrong with you, Erin? You're a junkie, an engaged junkie.*

We went around the circle and talked about how we felt during the last family group meeting. The other two women there were mothers. They cried for losing their womanhood to drugs and alcohol. They cried for the pain of failing their children. They cried for wasting the best years of their lives. I was glad I was not them. *I will never be a mother.*

I found it so hard to relate to the drinkers. Alcohol was something I could always take or leave. And, conversely, I felt the distance from everyone when they said, "Wow, heroin is the one thing I would never do."

It was my turn to talk. I talked about my feelings in an unemotional way. I spoke about my shame and guilt. I said I was disappointed in myself. I shared that I felt exposed and naked. I talked about my parents and about their anger and sadness. I felt disconnected from all of it, like I was narrating someone else's story. Then John said something that brought heat to the surface of my skin: "Well, I think you finally got their attention."

"I don't think I was looking for their attention," I said.

I felt tears. My face, then neck, then bosom became wet and salty with a slow but steady trickle. I couldn't breathe. I had spent years learning how to control myself, control my emotions, control feeling anything at all. I hated this. *I can't do this. I can't feel this.* Everything inside me was breaking apart. I was cracking open. I didn't know if I hated it, or it was a relief, and it was probably both.

When group was over, I rushed out the door, down the hall, through the living room, and out onto the porch. I couldn't get the cigarette in my mouth fast enough. I was dizzy. *The patches.* I sat down and put my head between my knees. Lunch came and went. I barely ate and what I did eat I threw up. Nothing wanted to stay in me anymore—not food, not drugs, not tears, not lies.

After lunch, we went for a walk, led by Patty, another counselor there. She was in her late fifties, sober for twenty-five years. She looked like a schoolteacher from *Little House on the Prairie.* Rob, Von, and I lit up cigarettes, and they told their drug stories. They were both crackheads. Rob was a burly white guy—like Bluto from *Popeye*—and worked in construction in Simi Valley. Von was from Sri Lanka. He was the kind of guy who managed to blend into the walls with politeness, and he came from a family who never imagined their only son would end up smoking crack. They reminded me of some weird druggy version of Lenny and Squiggy from *Laverne & Shirley.*

I tried keeping my distance from Andrew, as we rounded the bend toward the Forest Lawn cemetery, a sister cemetery to the one I'd driven by so many times. The counselors used all sorts of half-baked metaphors to link our little house at the end of the street to the cemetery next door: "Jails, institutions, and death. That's where you'll end up if you keep using. You're already here, in an institution. The cemetery is right next door, waiting for you." They explained this as a metaphor. I didn't want to be the one to point out that it was not really a metaphor.

I could feel Andrew looking at me. *You have enough problems, Erin.* As we entered the gates, we inched closer to the real reward of the walk: feeding the swans. There was a peaceful pond, filled with noble swans. It was truly pastoral. Green, so much green, it soothed me. It soothed everyone else, too. Looking at us, here with the swans, I wondered if anyone could tell that we were a bunch of addicts on a field trip.

Feeling dizzy again, I lay down on the grass and closed my eyes. I was confronted by a series of quick cuts, scene to scene, the disjointed moments that led me there—moments I ran from, moments I'd hidden. I couldn't take it, so I opened my eyes. The grass smelled fragrant, damp, hopeful. I forgot for just a minute where I was and who I had become. I couldn't remember the last time I'd lain down in the grass and really felt it, smelled it. I turned my head to the side and inhaled, hoping somehow the feeling of being renewed would stick. I'd been running for so long—running from people and places and emotions and the overwhelming desire to die. Now I just wanted to stay there on the grass.

Heroin kept me from killing myself. The thought sounded ridiculous in my head, but also entirely true.

It was time to go. I tried to stand up, but I was far too dizzy. Everyone gathered around and waited while I sat, once again, with my head between my knees. I sensed that my fellow shipwrecked comrades felt sorry for me. I was the baby. I was the heroin addict. Maybe I was the girl they wanted to save, to avoid having to confront themselves.

Back at the house, I asked Patty if I could lie down. I walked down the hall, past an open door. There was someone new—a woman—and she was sobbing during her intake interview. I put my head down and walked past into my somber little room, with the pale blue drapes and the bed with the plastic sheets. I took my blue Converse All Stars off and curled up into a ball. It was useless to close my eyes, so I didn't. The spider had not moved from its spot above the dresser. *Maybe it's always been there*, I thought. *Maybe it's a test, to see if I'm paying attention.* My mind drifted into an assortment of various conspiracy theories.

Patty interrupted, "It's time for group, Erin."

Time in that bungalow rolled on. My muscles grew fatigued from days of convulsions, contracting and tightening, helping to push the poison out of me. During my second week there, I got my period. I called my mom and asked her to bring me some tampons. Instead, she sent Vincent. He arrived shortly before the nightly meeting. Every night there was a twelve-step meeting in the living room of our little house. People came from the outside. It was like a breath of fresh air, of promise, that I would somehow make it out of there and live again. I had put on makeup and was sitting on the porch flirting with Andrew. When I saw Vincent walking up, I stiffened and put out my cigarette. He looked at me, and I knew he could sense my attraction to Andrew.

We walked silently to the main office so he could be signed in as a visitor and the staff could inspect my tampons.

"Can we talk outside?" he asked.

We sat awkwardly in chairs on the side of the bungalow.

"You are all dressed up."

"I just have lipstick on," I said.

"I don't think you should be here. I want you to come back to France with me. It's LA. It's bad for you."

"Vincent… I'm a heroin addict. I can't leave. I need help."

We sat in silence, and I watched old anger resurface behind his eyes and in the tight grip of his fingers on the white metal chair.

"I just don't understand why you put a needle in your arm. A fucking needle."

"You're never going to forgive me," I said.

"Yeah, I don't know if I can forgive you."

I looked down at the delicate ring on my left hand. I dragged my right index finger back and forth over the diamond and the sides of the band and pulled it off.

"Here," I said, grabbing his hand and placing the engagement ring in his palm. "I can't wear this. I can't do this. I am so sorry…for everything."

"Really? You are going to do this to me, here? Now?"

"I'm sorry, I have to go."

I got up, tried to hug his stiff body that remained seated, and walked back inside the bungalow.

That night during the twelve-step meeting, a woman spoke about her life before getting clean—about being a junkie, a sex worker, and eventually a bank robber. Listening to her story, I felt like I knew her; she was the bank robber mother I never had. I spoke with her after the meeting and asked her to be my sponsor.

The night staff arrived. They brought in a movie, *Anaconda*, for us to watch and some microwave popcorn. Andrew sat next to me, and we watched the movie, and he watched me, and I watched him watching me. After the movie, Von and Rob took it upon themselves to fill the sad, lonely hot tub behind the house with laundry detergent. It made a lot of bubbles, a ridiculous amount of bubbles. We laughed but the night staff was not amused. Andrew and I had one last smoke on the porch. On the way back to our rooms, he pulled me toward him in the hallway and kissed me, and I let him, and I kissed him back.

Back in my room, I washed my face and put on my sweats and lay on top of my bed, staring up at the spider. I closed my eyes and dreamed while awake. I saw myself like a fractured mirror, at all different ages—as a little girl, lost and scared and running from the monster she believed lived inside her. I wanted to take that little girl in my arms and tell her it wasn't her fault. That she didn't make herself a monster. That she could be, should be, loved. But I still wasn't completely sure if this was true, which broke my heart a little more.

I saw myself as a teenager, constantly on the run from everything. I wanted to grab that teenager's shoulders and tell her to slow down, tell her to stop, tell her to stay still. But I still wasn't sure if she was capable of that. And I saw myself as Vincent's fiancée, and as his ex-fiancée. *I did the right thing, didn't I? I had to let him go. I had to.* I felt the tears come. I hated feeling sorry for myself. *This is not me.* I shuffled out to the office to see if the night staff would let me have a smoke.

William was there in the office. He had the radio on and the faint sounds of "Groovin'" by The Young Rascals played. The song caught me in the throat, the way a piece of music can immediately make you feel nostalgia for some other time or place. William was a sixty-year-old black man from Oakland. He didn't get clean until he was forty-five. He was a junkie, too. He offered to join me on the porch for a smoke. He told me more of his story. He told me about being in gangs and selling dope and smuggling dope in jail and losing his wife and kids and never getting to say goodbye to his parents. He told me about hitting a bottom so low and getting clean and being grateful for his life today.

I thought about how much of his life, his story, was shaped by the color of his skin, by the place he was born, by the lack of access to all the things I had access to. The guilt for what I'd been given—for all that I'd taken for granted, for all that I'd squandered—lodged in my chest like an anchor of remorse. As he spoke, the tears came back. For the first time, the tears felt okay. The tears felt appropriate. The tears felt necessary.

"William, I feel so guilty. I feel so guilty."

He placed his hand on my shoulder and said, "You gotta stop blaming yourself for everything. You've been sick. But it's really gonna be okay, kid. You're gonna be okay."

I believed him. That heavy feeling in my chest began to dissolve, at least a little bit. Relief washed over my sore, stinky skin. I felt a calm I had not felt in years, maybe ever. There we sat, William and I, on the porch, on the last house at the end of the street, next to a cemetery, where I was learning to live again.

CHAPTER 12
Tap-Dancing Backward
October 1997

Like most treatment programs, my rehab set up an aftercare plan for me. In lieu of going from the bungalow into a sober living house, I made an agreement to live with my mom for sixty days. I attended outpatient group twice a week at the bungalow and committed to ninety twelve-step meetings in ninety days. I had a blueprint for how to get through these early days of sobriety, and I would need one. I still couldn't sleep well and days were long. But for once, I didn't feel so unmoored; I felt hopeful.

"Hi! Welcome!" a tall, skinny guy in his thirties said as he stuck out his hand to shake mine.

We were on the steps outside a building that resembled a log cabin in West Hollywood, set back from the street. I couldn't believe I'd never noticed it before. I was there for my first twelve-step meeting outside rehab, and I was nervous, and thankfully not alone. Tessa was with me.

Tessa and I met toward the end of my stay in rehab. She'd been attending their intensive outpatient program. She was five years older than me, a rock 'n' roll girl through and through, with long dark hair and a cool vibe, like she just stepped off Led Zeppelin's tour bus in the midseventies. She worked for a record label, and her boss sent her to treatment when he noticed that she was spinning out on alcohol and cocaine. She was my first real friend in sobriety.

The tall, skinny guy had a shaggy haircut and a broad smile, and as I shook his hand, he said, "I'm Bill."

"Hi, I'm Erin. You look so familiar."

We stood on the steps and chatted. Tessa and I told him that it was our first meeting outside rehab. As we made small talk, I suddenly realized how I knew him.

"Wait, Bill, did you used to live in Beachwood Canyon… and, um, did you by any chance used to sell drugs?"

He laughed and said, "Yup! Did I sell to you?"

"Oh my God! Yeah, well, not to me, but to this weird guy I was dating. Mike-Jim. He had a weird tic where he would compulsively clear his throat."

"Oh yeah! I think I remember him."

And with that, I made my second true friend after rehab.

Those early weeks outside rehab were filled with at least one twelve-step meeting a day, hours spent at Swingers diner on Beverly Boulevard drinking coffee and eating fries, killing time with Bill and Tessa, and sleeping with Andrew from rehab. That, however, didn't last long; Andrew relapsed, and I knew that I couldn't continue to be around him and not relapse. I cared for Andrew, but I cared for myself more and that was a first. I avoided thinking about Vincent too much by filling every minute of my day. I felt determined to stay sober. I started working again as a wardrobe stylist and diligently went through the twelve steps with my sponsor.

My first weekend at my mom's house, my dad came to town again to see me. I spent my Saturday afternoon with them both.

Dad was getting ready to leave, Mom was getting ready for a
blind date, and I was about to head to Tessa's. My cell phone
rang. It was Polly. She was crying, frantic, calling me from a
payphone at rehab. She'd been in treatment for four days, and
Milo was home alone.

"Erin, you have to go check on Milo," she said. "He's been
kicking at home, and he told me he couldn't do it. I'm scared
he's going to kill himself. Please."

"Oh God. Polly, I can't go there."

"Please, please. If you don't go, I'll have to leave. I can't stay
here and not help him."

"Hold on, okay?" I said as I set the phone down.

I went to find my parents in the kitchen. I told them that
Polly and Milo had been using, that Polly was in rehab, that
Milo was all alone, and that Polly wanted me to check on him.
I knew I couldn't do what she was asking me to do; if I did, I
knew Milo and I would get high.

My mom looked so pretty, ready for her date, leaning tall and
golden against the kitchen counter. She straightened up and said,
"You're not going. I'll go. We'll go."

Dad looked at her and back at me. "We'll go."

Mom called and canceled her blind date with the man who
would become my stepfather. I swelled with gratitude. That
they would do this for Milo, for me.

Later, my mom told me they found him in terrible shape—
frail and mortified. My mom told him not to be embarrassed,
that they were there to help. My dad went to the grocery store
for supplies. My mom cleaned him up, cleaned up the apartment,
cleaned the litter box and fed the cats. They made him mashed
potatoes and cut up bananas. They made him drink water and
tea, and my mom changed his sheets. My parents told me that
they had no choice but to go, that if it had been me—sick and
alone—they would have wanted someone else's parents to do
the same for me.

I hoped that Milo would make it through his kick and that Polly would finish her twenty-eight days and that we could go to meetings together and drink coffee and eat french fries at Swingers. Polly left rehab a couple of days later, and I didn't hear from either of them for a long time. It would be almost a decade before I'd see them again. As painful as it was to step away from a friendship that I'd had since I was a teenager, the part of me that wanted to survive held me back from reaching out.

One night at the twelve-step meeting, the floor was opened to anyone who wanted to share. A tall, lanky, handsome guy with messy golden hair and prominent cheekbones walked to the front of the room.

Tessa elbowed me and whispered, "He looks like the Hugo Boss model."

I didn't catch his name because I was paying attention to Tessa.

He stood at the podium and told a story about needing to make amends to his old neighbors because he'd stolen their dog when he was high. He did it because he thought they didn't take good care of the dog, but then the damn dog escaped, and no one ever saw the dog again. He had the whole room doubled over in laughter. I was smitten.

When we left the meeting, Tessa and I talked about "Dog Boy" and what a babe he was and "did he really steal that dog or was it a joke?" Every time I saw him at a meeting, I'd get nervous and sweaty and stay as far away from him as possible.

I wasn't prepared for the onslaught of men who would come into my orbit as a newly sober young woman. Addiction has an energy, an energy that still surges inside you as your body adjusts. When you take alcohol and drugs away, sex and love can become the brightest, shiniest, and seemingly safest place to put all that energy. I learned that I'd have to differentiate between who was genuinely being friendly and supportive from those who were only interested in sex with a fresh face on the sobri-

ety scene. And, it was a scene. Twelve-step meetings in the late
'90s in Los Angeles sometimes felt like singles bars without the
booze. In some ways, the vibrant socializing made it easy and
appealing to want to be there, but in other ways it served as a
veil from the fact that many of us were so sick.

I made a few friends outside Tessa and Bill, mostly men. I
found it harder to make friends with the women in the program.
One I did befriend was Sunny, a chatty and friendly Korean girl,
a few years older than me, with short blue hair. She grew up in
Beverly Hills, was going through a divorce, and like me, was a
little boy crazy without drugs.

One rainy Monday afternoon in January 1998, Bill and I
were thrift shopping at Wasteland on Melrose. We were talking
about crushes, and I had just confided in him that I had a huge
crush on Dog Boy, whose name I didn't even know. We turned
a corner around a rack of vintage leather jackets, and I quite lit-
erally ran into him. Dog Boy was standing right in front of me.

"Hey," he said. "I know you."

He knows me?

"Hi, what are you doing here?" *Oh my GOD; what a stupid
question.*

"Just looking around. Are you going to the meeting tonight?"
he asked, referring to the meeting in the log cabin building.

"Oh yeah."

"I'm Pete, by the way."

"Erin."

"I know. See you tonight," he said, and with that he headed
out the door.

Bill and I spent the next twenty minutes dissecting whether
he'd heard any of our conversation. I was half mortified and half
thrilled. *He knew my name.*

That night at the meeting, Pete and I chatted on the steps,
smoking. He was smoking Gitanes, which I'd smoked when I

lived in Paris. Afterward, he invited me to go with him and his friends to Swingers. We shared a Burst of Blue milkshake and some soggy fries, and he played "Torn and Frayed" by the Rolling Stones on the jukebox. When he talked, I found myself staring at his full lips and kind hazel eyes and crooked teeth. I loved his crooked teeth. I found out that we'd gotten sober one day apart. He was thirty-two, a photographer, and currently in a sober living house in West LA. At the end of the night, he asked for my number.

He called the next day and asked me out on a date. When we hung up, I leaped across my living room and danced around like I was twelve years old. *Could I really be falling for someone again?* Without drugs, I was left open, without my usual defenses. It felt scary and exhilarating and I wanted this new vulnerability as much as it terrified me. This didn't feel like a fling or a distraction, and I wasn't sure I was ready for it, but I couldn't stop myself from wanting all of it.

That Friday, Pete took me on our first date. We saw *LA Confidential* and ate ramen at a Japanese noodle house on the west side. He told me about his drug history and that he struggled with depression. He told me about moving to the US from the Netherlands when he was fourteen, about boarding school, and about losing his father to suicide. He was open and honest and I knew I could fall in love. It was raining, and when he drove me home, he parked in front of my building on Beachwood and we made out, listening to Morphine's *Cure for Pain* album. Warm and alone in his car, we made our own bubble. I wanted to stay forever.

In early sobriety, it's generally advised that you don't get into a relationship within the first year. It's not a shock I didn't listen. Pete and I became involved very quickly. I felt like he was my destiny. I adored him. He was warm and kind, and I was drawn to him like a magnet. As much as I'd loved Vincent, I never truly trusted him. I trusted Pete in a way I had not trusted men before. But I was petrified because I didn't trust myself.

A couple of months into my relationship with Pete, on a stormy Tuesday night, we went to a meeting together. As we were about to get into my car, I heard a woman's voice behind us shout, "Pete!"

It was his ex-girlfriend, Cynthia. They'd been together for seven years and had broken up before he got sober. He walked over to talk to her, and I got in the car, out of the rain. We were meeting friends at Highland Grounds, a coffeehouse, and now we were late. I sat there with a knot in my stomach as the rain pelted the windshield in an angry chorus. He got back in the car.

"What was that about?" I asked.

"I guess she tracked me down. She wants to talk to me. She wants closure."

"It's kind of stalker-ish, don't you think?"

"I guess. I need to talk to her. I need her to know there's no chance of us getting back together."

"Now?" I asked.

"Well, I kind of told her we were going to Highland Grounds, and she's coming there to talk."

"Are you serious?"

I felt tingly and flushed, and I wondered if he was telling me the whole story.

We got to Highland Grounds and met Bill and Sunny and some others at a large table in the corner. Pete looked nervous, and I was furious. Cynthia walked in and looked at our table, made eye contact with me, and glared. She was attractive, a bit older than him, and looked like my complete opposite—curvy, blonde, with a professional air about her.

They sat at the counter and talked for over an hour. Bill and Sunny did their best to keep me company. At one point, Sunny went to the counter under the guise of ordering something so she could eavesdrop. Cynthia was angry. She'd expected they'd get back together after he sobered up. And she was even angrier that he was dating a "twenty-four-year-old twit."

I felt humiliated. Technically, Pete hadn't done anything wrong or untrustworthy. He did give her closure that night, and she never showed up anywhere again. But I felt betrayed by her existence.

Later that week, I was at a late-night meeting on the roof of a rec center in West Hollywood with Bill. After the meeting, people would often hang around, chatting and smoking and drinking bad coffee. I was doing all those things in my leopard coat while sucking on a lollipop and furiously tap-dancing backward when Bill walked up with a tall, solid-looking guy with messy brown hair and said: "Erin, do you know Nate?"

"Hi," I said, sticking out my hand as I kept on tap-dancing backward.

"Hi," Nate said, and he watched me for a moment. "I have to say this is a fairly disarming way to meet someone. What are you doing?"

"Disarming?" I asked and laughed. "I'm tap-dancing. Sort of."

I was sober and hyper, and my skin could not contain me. He was large and steady like an anchor. I can't remember anything else about the meeting that night, because he had the darkest eyes and I fell into them trying to find my reflection.

Bill and Nate and I drove to the beach that night, and rope got caught on the axle underneath my car. Nate got right under it and undid the rope. Then we went to his apartment and watched a Richard Kern film. I left at 6:00 a.m. and he wanted to kiss me, and Bill told him I had a boyfriend, and he asked me why I didn't tell him, and I said, "Well, you never asked."

Nate's entry into my life revived my old pattern with romantic partners. I wouldn't leave Pete, but I stayed in Nate's orbit and brought him banana pancakes early in the morning from Duke's on Sunset. We'd lie in the grass outside his apartment and smell the eucalyptus tree in the courtyard. They made me think about when I was fourteen and Sam and I did the same thing before he died.

On one of those banana pancake mornings, we ate in his bed, and he traced my bony arm with his finger and asked, "Who are you and where did you come from?"

And I told him that I loved him, but I couldn't be with him, and we were both confused by that. He went down on me, and I touched him and then went home and felt horribly guilty. I climbed under the soft weight of my duvet and cried.

The truth was I loved him. The truth was I also loved Pete. When emotional intimacy becomes your greatest trigger, it feels impossible to sit still. I wanted both men to love me; I wanted to love both men. I couldn't bear being truly intimate with either one without some buffer. And that need was stronger than ever because my greatest emotional buffer—heroin—was gone.

Nate wrote me a love letter and said he couldn't see me. I ignored his request, and I went to see him anyway because I knew he wouldn't say no and he said, "You're incorrigible."

He said it more than once. And I was incorrigible, but I couldn't see myself clearly. I could only feel the need to smell him.

Then he left for San Francisco with another girl, and he relapsed, and his friends said it was my fault and I thought they were right. He left to go to Santa Fe, which was probably to get far away from me, but he wrote me letters. I read them and kept them under the mat in the trunk of my car.

I shut the door on Nate. Pete moved in and I started to panic. Once again, I craved the emotional intimacy I knew I could have with Pete, but every part of me wanted to destroy it and push it away. I missed disconnection. I missed being able to compartmentalize. I missed heroin.

CHAPTER 13
Curtain Call
August 1998

"Hi, Diana, it's me. You up? Can I come over?"

I had to clear my dry throat three times to get the words out. It was a hot late-August morning. Pete had already left for work, and I knew the moment my mind rattled awake what I wanted to do.

I had been using again for a couple of weeks—chipping, controlling how much and how often; I wasn't strung out yet. In the weeks since Pete had moved in with me and I'd shut the door on Nate, I'd started having panic attacks again—hot and sweaty and out of air. One afternoon I found myself walking into a boutique on Melrose where my friend Diana worked, just to see if she was there. I hadn't seen her, hadn't seen anyone I'd used with, for over ten months. Her pupils were pinned; I could tell she was high. After catching up on the changes in our lives, I asked her.

"Diana, are you high?"

She couldn't lie to me. And she refused to give me any. But I went back to the boutique again the next day, under the guise of bringing her lunch. I told her I was fine, and I told her that if she didn't give me any, I'd go downtown and score myself. Just like that, heroin was back in my life.

Every time I started using heroin again, it didn't feel like a consequential decision. I realize this is not a satisfactory answer for most people. The critical thing to understand about addiction is that my decision to get high, to get low, to exit, had been made long before the drug entered my body. Those triggers—the ones that came to life when my heart was open, when people got too close, when I felt myself vulnerable with others—woke up my primal defense, my addiction. That addiction lay dormant inside me, waiting, and would take over and let me believe the lie that using heroin wasn't a big deal. *I could get high. It didn't matter. No one would find out. We could pretend it never happened.* In all honesty, I didn't want to get high; I wanted to get unconscious. I wanted everything to shut down.

Now with Pete, I was at the inevitable point in my relationship when I desperately needed to escape. It was too much; I felt too much, I needed him too much, he expected too much. *Oh, Pete, I'm sorry for leaving you for so long.*

Diana was the only one I was getting high with because it would have shattered me if anyone else knew. I was sure it would shatter them, too. I was supposed to have been eleven months clean. Diana had been my way back in, but I refused to let my use become more widespread. The one thing I'd always felt certain about in my friendship with Diana was that she never judged me. I adored her for that, but my addiction exploited this kindness. Heroin had taken control of me again, the minute I'd manipulated Diana into giving me dope. As I threw on my jeans and T-shirt, I was already disconnecting from Pete, from my life, from my body. I had to disconnect or the shame would burn me up. I shook it off and headed to Diana's.

The air was heavy. With my air-conditioning blasting, I rolled down my window so I could smoke. What should have been a five-minute drive to Diana's place, two miles away, took twenty. The traffic made me anxious, and my stomach cramped up.

Diana lived off Hollywood Boulevard. The parking was scarce, and the last thing I felt like doing was fighting a tourist for a parking spot. I circled for fifteen minutes, my stomach continuing to curl into a ball, tight and hard. Finally, a spot. Cursing myself for wearing jeans, I was in a full sweat by the time I finished the two-block walk to her building.

Diana's apartment was a welcome respite from the oppressive heat and smog outside. She opened the door wearing, of course, a vintage slip and her fuzzy slippers. It was her uniform—much like it had been mine—when we got high, which was becoming increasingly frequent again. Diana looked so tiny to me, like a little witch with her long black hair and her crooked nose. She's very pretty and petite, and I have always felt like a giant next to her. The cool air of her apartment swept me in. Cigarettes, Nag Champa incense, her vanilla perfume, and the faintest undercurrent of Mexican black tar heroin swirled in the air around me.

The smell of dope always made me gag a little. It looks and smells like shoe polish and vinegar and something sweet that has turned a little rotten. It's not white and powdery, the kind you find in the Midwest and on the East Coast. The West Coast dealers primarily get dope from Mexico, and it's this black sticky tar-like substance, probably cut with something awful.

Diana's apartment was an incongruent blend of its 1960s prefab structure and her penchant for goth decor. The air-conditioning was always blasting; the shades were always drawn. I glanced at the television. She had been watching *The Craft*, starring Fairuza Balk and her teenage witch posse. We paused for a minute in the living room. Diana switched off the TV and turned on some music. Her cats eyed me from the corner. They knew too much. There was something about their side-eyed observation that made me nervous. I couldn't look at them.

Like a good friend, Diana had already cooked up and had needles ready for us. Walking down the long hallway to the bathroom, my body surged again with the overwhelming need to disconnect. I peed and then proceeded to fix. It wasn't a particularly large hit, but the second I took the syringe out of my left arm, relief and warmth flooded through me, knocking me back. Somewhere in the dimmest edge of my mind, I wondered why it was hitting me so hard. The taste coated the back of my throat and the roof of my mouth. That familiar taste, somewhere between rubbing alcohol and burnt sugar, made me queasy.

"I'm gonna go lie down," I said, or I think I said, but maybe I said nothing.

Her room felt even cooler and darker than the rest of the apartment. I had trouble focusing my eyes. The only thing that came into view was a painting of Ophelia that hung above the bed. I remained fixed on the painting until I lay down.

And I fell. The bed became a dark cloud, and I sank—slowly, deeper and deeper. This is what I was looking for. I wanted something more than asleep. I wanted to be comatose. I wanted my brain to stop, to completely stop. Descending, I recited a line over and over in my mind, *A woman is dragging her shadow in a circle*. I couldn't place it. I thought it might be Plath, but I kept losing the thought until I recited the line again.

Dimly aware of the sounds around me—the air-conditioning, the music from the other room—I drifted through a viscous sea of thought. The thoughts became too incoherent to hold on to, but the one image that kept returning was Hamlet's Ophelia drowning. I felt like Ophelia—sinking, half-insane, surrendering to some version of death. Sometimes I would meditate on that image, but then I would drift again, until those thoughts got smaller, fainter, further away.

I could stay here forever. The thoughts became dormant. My brain was silent; I was suspended. Occasionally, a sharp but distant sound interrupted the quiet. The sound clawed its way in. It made me aware of how vast this darkness was. Slight, and then bigger, chills slid over me, making me feel uneasy in the still and boundless black.

The faraway sound became more frequent, annoying like a buzzing fly. I wondered if the sound was coming from me. Suddenly, I felt sucked out of the darkness for the briefest moment. A curtain, in front of my face, opened, for a second at most. Light and sound flooded in, jarring me, but I fell back into the inert black pool. Then the curtains opened again, for a few seconds this time, jolting me. Back into darkness, I felt more and more annoyed by the interruption. I recited the line in my head, *A woman is dragging her shadow in a circle.*

The curtains opened once more, and I realized that the faraway sound was right in front of my face. It was coming from Diana. She was crying, screaming at me, shaking me. I drifted out of my body and saw her on the bed, practically on top of me, violently trying to get me to wake up. The darkness pulled me back in, and I felt calm. The curtains ripped open. I was angry.

"I'm just lying down for a minute. Leave me alone."

She didn't seem to hear me. Wasn't I shouting? Despite my efforts, no words came out. I held on to the black world—tried to remain there. The curtains opened, and I jerked my body up.

"What the fuck is your problem?" I screamed.

"Oh God, Erin, Erin, get up, get up! You weren't breathing," she choked out through tears.

I repeated myself, "What the fuck is your problem? I was just lying down for a minute."

Struggling to get up, I realized that the bed was soaked. I felt like I couldn't walk. My movements were stiff, jerky, uncontrolled. Completely disoriented, I swung my arm around and accidentally hit her in the face. I made my way to the bathroom. It felt like forever in that incredibly long hallway, slamming into walls, unable to get my balance. When I finally made it, I looked in the mirror. My face was icy gray and my lips were blue. They were blue. Blue. Confusion and dread set in as I realized that I had overdosed. I began to fall out of consciousness again.

Diana hoisted me into the shower. It must have looked comical. Little Diana, five-two and one hundred pounds soaking wet, trying to commandeer her friend who was six inches taller. She turned the water on and it ripped over my skin. I looked over at her, still only half processing what had just happened. She could hardly breathe as she slumped on the floor next to the shower, recovering. I was somewhere between the sensations of extreme numbness from the drug and the sharpness of the water on my skin. Ten minutes later, I stood up from the floor of the shower, turned the water off, tore off my wet clothes, and wrapped myself in a towel. Diana looked traumatized.

Still, none of it felt real. I held on to the stubborn thought that she overreacted. We walked back into the bedroom and surveyed the damage. Liquid had emptied out of my body all over her bed. I bent over and smelled it. It wasn't urine. I didn't know what it was.

"I thought you were dead," she whispered, "You weren't breathing, Erin. You were fucking blue."

She began to cry again. I looked at her and felt nothing, but I knew I had to say something.

"I'm sorry… I'm sorry I hit you. I was confused."

My lack of sincerity burned on my tongue and I wondered if I had in fact spoken. She continued crying, sitting on the floor.

"I can't get high with you anymore," she said.

"Okay." After the smallest of pauses: "Can I borrow some clothes, so I can get home?"

She gave me some shorts and a T-shirt. I gathered my still-soaked clothes that I was wearing earlier and prepared to leave.

"I'm really sorry, Diana. I'll call you later."

I had nothing else to say. And so, I headed back out into the oppressive heat. I felt shaky and kept pushing away the visual of my icy gray face and my blue lips staring back at me in Diana's mirror. I still needed an exit. It was barely midday. I had just enough time to score and get back to numb before Pete got home. There was no point in fighting it. Heroin was winning.

CHAPTER 14
Soggy Pancakes
March 2000

"I don't even want to go anymore," I said, crossing my arms and sighing.

"Well, I told Travis we were coming and either way we're going to be stuck in traffic."

I looked out the passenger window at the endless lines of cars all around us. The rain was starting to pick up. It was Sunday morning. Pete and I were stuck in LA marathon traffic on Franklin Avenue. Neither of us had remembered that the marathon was even happening. The distance from our apartment in Beachwood Canyon to the little diner on Sunset was around a mile, but we'd been trapped for over an hour, stopping and inching along, past the Bourgeois Pig, past Gelson's Market.

I felt like we were running out of air in the car. I could barely look Pete in the eye.

For the past year and a half, I'd been in a seemingly never-ending cycle of relapsing, hiding it, kicking, relapsing, hiding it, kicking. Pete had struggled, too, with his gambling and occasionally cocaine. I played the part of the understanding girlfriend, all the while smoking heroin in my car, in gas station bathrooms, and using off and on with Diana. After I'd overdosed that August afternoon with Diana, she and I took a break from using together, but it was short-lived. She was terrified after that episode that I'd overdose and die. Oddly, that fear was what reunited us. If we were getting high together, she could make sure I wasn't shooting up, only smoking heroin. She made me promise. I needed her; I needed someone to keep me from falling too far. I never used a needle again, and neither did she. I didn't want anyone to find me blue and close to death the way Diana had. And despite how many times I'd wanted to not exist, getting that close to dying scared me, too.

But now I was sober; I felt like I was losing my mind.

Just after Christmas, before the new millennium, I had relapsed again and this time Pete found out. For two weeks, we used together. And we stopped together. We got meds from a detox doctor and started going to twelve-step meetings again. Much like with all my other relapses, I didn't tell anyone else. I pretended I'd been sober all along.

I'd recently gone back to therapy. Karen was a warm and generous therapist—who felt more like a favorite aunt than a clinician—with wild auburn curls and chunky necklaces. Pete and I were seeing her, separately and together. We were both struggling with depression and our own past traumas. As comfortable as I was with Karen, I didn't tell her about any of the many relapses. I rationalized that they were short-lived and unimportant, but I still carried them with me and internalized them as failings.

The relapses did matter. The more I lied, whether through words or omission, the stronger the shame inside me became. It's one of the most challenging parts of long-term recovery from drugs. The people who love you, even others in recovery, can unwittingly place expectations on you. The truth is relapse, while not a requirement, is a very common part of the recovery process. And it is just that—a process. I became fixated, like I had with grades and horseback riding and socializing growing up, on recovering the right way. I *had* to do it right. I had to be a good girl. I had to prove I was lovable. When I didn't or couldn't, the shame emerged like a spiral virus, each slip leading me further down, further in, making it that much harder to find my way out.

In January, after Pete and I had sobered up, my highs and lows escalated. Pete could see it. Karen could see it. I began opening up to both of them about my past sexual abuse. Karen referred me to a new psychiatrist. I'd tried going on medications over the past couple of years. Some of them made me feel worse. Wellbutrin had worked for me, but every time it worked, I thought I didn't need it anymore, so I would stop. And I felt tremendous shame over needing medication. I worried it meant I wasn't sober. I wanted what was wrong with me to be that I was a junkie. I could face that. I couldn't face the possibility that I was even more broken, that I was mentally ill.

On my second appointment to the psychiatrist, my mom wanted to come with me. She wanted to be supportive. My relationship with my mom had steadily improved over the past couple of years. The man she'd had the blind date with, on the night she and Dad helped Milo, had become my stepfather, and my mom had never been more stable. She was happy and healthy, and it was a relief. My stepdad—tall, athletic, kind, and steady— was a doctor, and he brought normalcy to our lives.

The psychiatrist's office was deep in the Valley, in an unassuming white office building, where every door looked the same, and you had to squint to check the nameplates. We sat across from the psychiatrist, my mom and I. I'd given him permission to explain what was going on with me and what combination of medication we would try.

"Given Erin's drug history and PTSD, some of what this looks

like is borderline personality disorder, but it may just be a combination of these other factors."

"Well, what do you mean by PTSD?" my mom asked.

The air stopped moving and I felt my pulse start to race.

"PTSD is very common, even expected, in individuals who
experienced sexual abuse, especially when it occurs at such a
young age."

My mom blanched and stiffened in her seat, a shocked expression glossed over her high cheekbones, and she said, "Well,
we don't really know if that happened."

I dissolved into the hard chair and the speckled linoleum floor
and the window with the crooked blinds and outside into the
setting sun behind us. The doctor responded to my mom, but
I couldn't hear what he said. My ears rang loudly—maybe they
were protecting me—blotting out every sound in the room.

If I spoke on the ride home, I don't remember it. I held the
prescription he'd written in my hands and tore tiny little pieces
off and placed them in my coat pocket like bread crumbs until
there was nothing left.

I hugged my mom goodbye, got out of the car, and walked up
the steps of Monroe Manor. I walked into my dark apartment, into
the kitchen, and got a box cutter out of the utility drawer. Then,
I stripped off my clothes, got into bed with the box cutter, and
curled into the fetal position and cried. After some time passed, I
heard the front door open and Pete's footsteps.

"Erin?"

I couldn't answer. He sat on the bed and lightly touched my
back, and I shivered. He took me in his arms and held me while
I sobbed.

"What is it?" he asked. "Did something happen?"

I couldn't speak. I could barely catch my breath between the
snot and the tears and my shaking body.

"Please," I said. "Just leave me alone."

I felt embarrassed and ashamed. I wanted him out of the room.

I wanted it to stop; like always, I just wanted everything to stop. I couldn't get out of the circular thought that this was all I ever wanted. *Stop. Stop. Stop.*

Alone again in the room, the tears did stop, and I took that box cutter and began jabbing myself in the leg, gently at first— like a gathering of raindrops trying to penetrate my skin—and then with more force until I started carving small sections of my thigh in little circles. Pete suddenly appeared next to the bed. He came back in, alarmed by the silence.

"Erin, what are you doing?"

He grabbed for the box cutter, but I wouldn't let go, I kept it jammed into my leg. He wrestled it away from me.

"Please, please, I just want it to stop," I said.

Pete picked me up and wrapped me in a sheet and held me like a child. He made me drink water, put a T-shirt and underwear on me, and cleaned up my leg and put Neosporin and Band-Aids in open places. I hadn't gone very deep with any of my cuts.

"How could you possibly love me?" I asked.

He kissed my forehead and told me he loved me.

I fell asleep for a little while and woke up to hear Pete talking to someone on the phone in the living room. I strained to hear, and I crept out of bed and sat on the floor next to the door. He was talking about a "plan" for me, about telling my parents, and getting me into treatment at Sierra Tucson. *I am not going into crazy person treatment.* I stood up and walked into the living room.

"Hi," I said.

Pete looked up from the couch with his kind hazel eyes.

"Hi," he said. "Sunny, I have to call you back."

He set down the phone, and I straightened up, doing my best to appear pulled together as I stood there in a T-shirt and un-derwear and Band-Aids on my leg.

"Please, please, don't tell my parents."

"Erin, I don't know. I… You scared me. I want you to get help."

"I'm okay. I swear. I just had a really shitty time with my mom at the psychiatrist. She, like, doesn't believe that I have any reason to be so fucked up."

Pete looked at me and I knew he understood. He got up and wrapped his arms around me, resting his chin on my shoulder. He whispered in my ear, "I believe you."

I promised Pete I'd start medication and promised to keep going to therapy and more twelve-step meetings and to throw away the box cutter. I did some of these things, but that night I also began to build a wall between us. He had seen too much, he knew too much, he cared too much, and I resented him for all the vulnerability I felt.

In February, I started a new job to give me some stability at a boutique that had just opened up on Sunset Plaza. CeCe, my new boss, had moved to LA from New York to open the store. We became fast friends. She was petite and thin and bronzed with sharp cheekbones and green eyes. She was glamorous and fun, and I wanted to be like her—thinner, sharper, more fun. The more time I spent with her, the less connected I felt to Pete. He never wanted to go out. *I'm young; I want to have fun*, I thought. *I don't want to be stuck here in this apartment thinking about what's wrong with me.*

Around the same time, I met Jack. Jack was a drummer, a fading rock star whose career had turned south because of his drug use. When I met him, he was sober and funny—God, he was so funny—and his extroverted personality was the opposite of Pete's. I found myself getting excited about seeing him at meetings and thinking about him when I woke up. He was new and fresh, and he hadn't seen all the horrible parts of me that Pete had.

I felt pulled again toward two futures—one with Pete, who knew my darkest secrets and loved me anyway, and one with Jack, who knew nothing but the light parts I'd shown him. I wondered if things could be different with Jack, if I could reinvent myself once again and leave all my mess behind me.

★ ★ ★

The car behind us laid on the horn.

"Where does he want me to go?" Pete said.

I sighed again, loudly, over the squeaky sound of the windshield wipers, and Pete turned toward me.

"What?"

"What?" I asked back.

"What's going on with you?"

"I don't know. I just feel. Uck, I just feel fucking trapped in this car right now."

We sat in silence for a moment.

"Pete… I don't know if I can… I feel like maybe we should take a break."

I looked at him, and he swallowed hard and stared straight ahead at the traffic in front of us.

"A break."

"Yeah, I mean. I don't know. I just feel like you're mad at me all the time because I want to go out and I'm mad at you because you don't."

"I can't do a break. If you… If that's what you need, then we should just break up. But know this—if we break up, that's it. We are not getting back together. I'm not going to play that game with you."

We sat in silence again, and I wondered what it would feel like in that car if Jack was sitting in the driver's seat, with his sparkly blue eyes and mischievous smile. We finally made it past Western and traffic opened up.

We got to the diner and Travis and his girlfriend were there waiting for us. I did my best to pretend we hadn't just talked about breaking up in the car, but I looked across the table at Pete and could see the hurt in his eyes. The waitress set down my breakfast in front of me and two large teardrops fell onto the stack of golden pancakes. I cut them up and put too much maple syrup on them, and pretended to eat, but just moved pieces around on the plate, making pancake soup, trying to keep up with the conversations at the table.

I wondered how different things would have been if we'd bought that loft in Providence. In November, we went to see my dad in Rhode Island and we talked about getting married; I looked at rings. We talked about getting out of LA. My dad wanted to help me buy something, a little piece of material happiness, make a path for me, again. We looked at a townhouse on Benefit Street near Brown that had a darkroom in the basement but was way too much house for us. Then we found a loft—a raw space with exposed brick and views of the water near my favorite Italian restaurant. There were multiple offers and we didn't get it. When we got back to LA, I started looking at condos and lofts, resigned to be in a city that I didn't care for.

When we got back in the car, I felt sick and panicky. I loved Pete. I did. It was me I wanted to dump.

"Pete, I don't want to break up. I'm sorry. It's just been a tough couple of months. I love you."

He started the car and leaned over and kissed me.

"I love you, too."

Days later, I hung out with Jack after a meeting. We went back to his apartment and talked and smoked and laughed.

"You're such a Zingo," he said.

"A Zingo?"

"Yes."

I laughed, "Is that a good thing?"

"Yes. You're adorable," he said.

Then he leaned toward me and kissed me.

"I have to go," I said.

He walked me to my car and we stood there kissing for a long time. I came home at 3:00 a.m. with burning lips. Pete was in bed, awake, angry in the quiet way he got angry.

"Where were you?"

"Out. With friends. We got something to eat and hung out," I said.

"Until 3:00 a.m.?"

"Yeah."

We lay in silence for minutes that felt like hours and I said, "Pete, I think we have to take a break. I'm not happy. I love you but I'm not happy."

"You'd better be sure this is really what you want because once it's done, it's done."

It was the same thing he'd said to me the week before.

"I'm sure," I said, but I wasn't.

CHAPTER 15
Blood Moon
October 2000

Oh God. I'd peed on my hand. *Why are you so nervous? There's no way you could be pregnant. But I'm never late. You're not that late.* My hand trembled as the voices in my head debated fertility. My fertility. *I don't want children. I've never wanted children. I can't even take care of myself. The world is overpopulated.* This was my mantra on motherhood.

My hand shook as I held the stick swathed in toilet paper. I hated smoking inside, but I lit a cigarette anyway, put the lid down, and sat on the toilet. And I waited. I faced myself in the long mirror in front of me. My eyes looked tired, burdened. My short, choppy hair was getting too long. The last time I went to Berto to get my hair cut, I ran into Pete. *What are the odds?* Pete had been getting his hair cut by Berto for years; I felt like I should relinquish him. More important, seeing Berto reminded me of what I lost or, more precisely, what I gave up, even though I ran into Pete all the time, all over the place.

I was vaguely nauseous, but that wasn't a sign of anything; it was my status quo. Inhale, blow. I didn't have an ashtray and ashed into my hand, but the ashes fell because I was still holding the stick. Standing up, I opened the lid, threw the cigarette in the toilet, put the stick in the back pocket of my jeans, and washed my hands. I could see the cup out of the corner of my eye.

I felt so stupid; I wasn't supposed to pee *on* the stick, I was supposed to pee in the cup and dip the stick. Grabbing the directions, I realized this was not my only mistake.

"Place the test stick on a flat surface with the windows facing up for at least two minutes. If you wish, replace the cap to cover the absorbent tip."

I threw the evidence into the trash can and covered it with a wad of toilet paper. It could wait. *I'm sure I'm not pregnant anyway.*

Night came, and I told Jack nothing. There was nothing to tell. He fell asleep watching *Law & Order.* We weren't officially living together, but he was with me all the time. Earlier that spring, right after my breakup with Pete, my dad bought me a condo in Hollywood on Franklin, just west of La Brea. It didn't feel like home. A part of me felt I didn't deserve it, like so much of what I was given. The building was nice and had great amenities. But my apartment felt haunted—and I was the one who brought the ghosts.

I slipped out to go to Rite Aid. It was midnight, there was a blood moon in the sky, and the Rite Aid on the corner of Fairfax and Sunset was populated with its usual mix of night crawlers. Before I could get out of my car, a homeless man knocked on my window. I opened the door and handed him some change. He looked at it and back up at me with watery eyes, but said nothing. A group of trans sex workers, congregating in the corner of the parking lot, laughed loudly and suddenly. It startled me. I saw a blonde woman in a wheelchair by the entrance, doing leg lifts. *Is that Francine Dancer?* Francine had a show on public-access television; she'd dance around in a bikini. I saw her everywhere, in her wheelchair, moving it along with her feet, like Fred Flintstone's car. She was always wearing something skimpy with platforms, and lipstick smeared across her face. We didn't know each other, but I saw her so often, I greeted her anyway.

"Hi, Francine."

She looked at me, wide-eyed, then past me, and said, "Hi, sugar!"

Inside, it was too bright. The Rite Aid glare was stifling. *Why am I here?* I grabbed two bags of Halloween candy—Kit Kats and Reese's Peanut Butter Cups—but changed my mind, put them back, and got Butterfingers and York Peppermint Patties.

A trans woman in a purple miniskirt and matching eye shadow stood next to me, smiling. "I always wondered who the hell bought Yorks."

I nodded and she laughed. She kept laughing; I stopped by the feminine hygiene aisle, grabbing another EPT test, a hopeful box of tampons, and some condoms. *Going off of the pill was beyond stupid.* As I walked to my car, Francine said, "Bye, sugar!" I waved without turning around.

I opened my apartment door and stepped into the dark living room. Jack was still asleep on the couch. On my way to the balcony, I grabbed a blanket and placed it over him. He was smiling in his sleep. The light from the window made his pale face glow, and in an uncharacteristic moment of tenderness, I brushed his black hair off his forehead. In the six and half months we'd been together, Jack and I had a blast. He was all the fun and high energy I was missing from Pete. We made each other laugh, we were sexually compatible, and he brought out my musical side, teaching me how to play guitar. Even so, my heart was at a safe, remote distance. It was still with Pete.

I sat on the balcony, facing the Hollywood Hills, and smoked and ate candy and pretended to ignore the nausea. It felt colder than usual that October. Octobers in LA are usually hot and dry, the epitome of "earthquake weather." That year there was a constant chill; I felt it on the back of my neck.

The next morning, I was up way too early. I don't think I

slept at all. I headed to the bathroom, grabbed the test from underneath the sink, peed in the cup, dipped the stick, and waited. I felt a little crampy and was optimistic about my period. Five minutes passed, and I looked at the stick. There were two lines in the window.

The blood drained fast and hard from my head to my feet. *Wait, what does that mean?* I grabbed the instructions and read. "Two lines indicate a positive result."

Positive? *Positive.* This result was anything but positive. I sat on the floor and lit a cigarette. My face was going numb. I stopped breathing.

Action. I needed to take action. *Do I call my ob-gyn? I can't. I don't want him to know.* I got dressed. Sitting at the computer, I searched for abortion clinics in Los Angeles. Scrolling through antiabortion sites and family planning clinics, I found a private doctor in Beverly Hills, and I wrote the number on the corner of an envelope, which I ripped off and shoved in my pocket.

I heard Jack stirring on the couch behind me. I quickly shut off my computer and went back out on the balcony. I couldn't look at him just then.

I waited and waited for Jack to leave the condo. This took a while because he didn't have anywhere to go. He was holding on to his former self, the self that was a rock star, the self that toured and made money doing what he loved, the self that lived high and glamorous until he flushed it down the toilet with heroin. What did he have, a year clean? *He would make a terrible father. I would make an even worse mother.* I was hanging on to my sobriety by a very bare thread.

Finally, he left to meet someone for coffee. I made the call. There were no appointments until the following Tuesday. That was five days away. The woman on the phone explained that when I came in, they would give me a test to confirm the pregnancy. Then the doctor would discuss the "procedure" with me, and if I was ready to take the next step, I'd be put under "twilight" sedation for the "procedure." She also told me I needed someone to drive me home. I hung up the phone. I didn't know what to do with myself, but I knew I wanted to get high.

I'd been sober since January, when I was still with Pete, with the exception of a two-day relapse in May to mask the pain I was feeling from our breakup. I'd told no one about that relapse. Now here I was again, inching toward what felt like an inevitability.

I got onto the giant Indonesian daybed in my living room, pulled a cashmere throw over me, and turned on the television. Mindlessly flipping through channels, I thought back to just a couple weeks prior when I was with Jack and CeCe in Chicago, visiting Jack's parents. CeCe and Jack had come into my life at the same time and the three of us had been inseparable that summer. We all went to see Godspeed You! Black Emperor play one night. It was magical. We watched from backstage, practically sitting on the stage with the band. There must have been upward of twenty musicians up there.

When we left the theater, it was snowing. We drove along Lake Michigan and all the way up into Evanston and past Northwestern University.

Driving past the college campus made me think about how I'd never finished school and I missed it. Being a good student was something I knew how to do, it was an identity I could wear. I decided that night I wanted to go back to school, and when we got back to Los Angeles, I'd made some calls and found out I could reenroll at USC for the spring semester. Now I was crying on my daybed on a Thursday afternoon—pregnant, feeling on the precipice of self-destruction. I'd felt this way before, every time I relapsed, when all reasoning in my brain was no match for my need to *leave*.

The next few days I continued to say nothing. But Sunday came, and I couldn't be alone with my pregnancy anymore. Jack was drinking his second cup of coffee, wrapping up a call with his mom. I watched him on the phone, walking in circles around the room, nodding as he spoke, oblivious to what I was about to tell him. I could picture his mom's sweet Irish accent on the other end, always tinged with a bit of worry. *Was Jack being a good boy?* He was a thirty-six-year-old man, but he still wanted to be a good boy, and he rarely was. I understood his plight.

He set his cell phone down.

"I'm pregnant."

"What?"

"I'm pregnant."

"What do you mean, you're pregnant? No, you're not pregnant. You're a hypochondriac."

"It's not a disease... I took a test."

He grabbed his cigarettes, lit one, and began pacing, smoking and running his hands through his hair over and over.

"I mean, I just can't deal with this right now. I can barely afford to take care of myself. I just can't believe this. Why didn't you warn me?"

"Warn you? Warn you how?"

Whenever Jack got hyper like this, the more still I became. His nervous energy turned me to stone.

"I made an appointment."

He looked at me, bewildered.

"For an abortion."

"Oh, thank God," he said, blowing smoke into the living room. He didn't offer to pay.

"I don't think I want you to go with me. Can you please smoke outside?"

He responded by retreating to the balcony with his coffee and cigarette. I went into my bedroom and shut the door.

Later that morning, we went to an AA meeting. During the break, I walked to the back of the rec center to smoke. I needed some space. Jill was there, a woman I knew from meetings. We weren't particularly close but I liked her. While we smoked and chatted and her long black hair waved in the breeze, I told her I was pregnant. And I told her I made an appointment. And she told me she would be taking me on Tuesday. And I said okay. This type of gesture, of being there for someone you hardly knew, was prevalent in the twelve-step community. It's a major part of why twelve-step programs can be so helpful, especially in early sobriety. I wish I had leaned on that community more. Most of the time, I did what I'd always done, acted like I had it all together, all the time.

Monday morning, I woke up with heaviness bearing down on me—a weight made of all the things I didn't want to confront. It lay there like a lead blanket on my chest. I found myself gasping for air and trying to talk myself out of a panic attack.

I went for a drive. I drove right into the Valley, into North Hollywood. I drove right up to Juan's; I walked up to the door and knocked. He answered, holding his baby girl.

"Ehhhh, long time. You don't call me. You don't love me no more?"

"Oh, you know, I've been traveling and stuff."

"Well, come on, *chica*."

I could feel the sweat under my arms the second I stepped through his door. My body knew what was coming. I hoped I wouldn't have to make small talk for too long. Juan could be chatty, and he loved nothing more than having *chicas* around to talk to about his relationship problems and the baby and his girlfriend and his truck and his wife back in Mexico.

I looked at him and held up four fingers.

"Here, you take Jazmin," he said, thrusting the baby toward me, so he could go to the bedroom and get the drugs.

I held her with stiff arms, afraid I might drop her, afraid she might know there was a baby inside me. *There is no baby. You would be a terrible mother.* I paced back and forth and then walked to the hallway so I could keep talking to Juan from the other side of the bedroom door and stop looking into Jazmin's big almond-shaped brown eyes.

"Where's Vanessa?" I asked.

"Oh shit. She's mad at me again. What's new. She's across the street at her mom's."

He returned, took Jazmin back, and motioned for me to sit. He put her in the playpen and then sat next to me, took my hand, and dropped four blue balloons the size of marbles in it.

"Thanks," I said, handing him $80. I stood up and wobbled a little.

"You leaving already?"

"Yeah, I have to meet my boyfriend."

"Okay, *chica*."

He stood up and hugged me. Juan treated me like his favorite niece—his favorite niece who gave him thousands of dollars for heroin.

"Tell Vanessa I said hi."

Feeling shaky on the way home, and once again vaguely nauseous, I drove through McDonald's and got myself a chocolate milkshake. My jeans were hot, and not wanting the balloons of tar heroin to melt, I took them out of my pocket. I parked my car in the McDonald's parking lot on Sunset Boulevard and considered throwing the balloons away. My next thought was how I could get Jack to leave, so I could be alone, just me and the drugs, and then I remembered that I'd sent him back to his apartment after the meeting the day before. It was the first night he'd spent in his own apartment in four months. I got out of the car, walked over to the trash can, and tossed the milkshake.

Walking in my front door, the empty quiet in my apartment filled me with relief. *I should put that on my gratitude list.*

I crouched on the bathroom floor, with my back against the door, even though I was alone. My sweaty fingers struggled to undo the knot in one of the blue balloons. I put the knot in my mouth and loosened it with my teeth. My hands shook as

I unwrapped the plastic wrap around the black tar heroin. The ringing in my ears got louder and vibrated through my body. That's how relapses always felt, like an electric field was buzzing all around me, pressing in on me until I broke.

I tore off a jagged piece of aluminum foil and ripped it into two. One piece got wrapped around a pen to make my straw and the other piece I turned into an imperfect square. I pressed a piece of tar into the foil square, lit the bottom up with a lighter, and inhaled.

I gagged from the first hit, and I spit into the toilet. I went back for a second and a third and then finally, the cloud that heroin brings began to float down over me. It erased that electric pressure, leaving its murky residue around my head like a cushion against thoughts.

It was a temporary cure. Not in the way I wanted it to, not the way it used to. I had a flash of a thought that maybe heroin just didn't work for me anymore. I'd heard this from other heroin users, that at a certain point it stops working in the same way it once did. Nonetheless, it dulled the feelings scraping around inside me.

Shame is a gatekeeper. Shame takes old shame and turns it into a new shame. The heroin helped push the guilt to the side. The grief I couldn't acknowledge stayed buried underneath, pulsating but muzzled, like a drugged dog. The high coated me with enough apathy to make it through the night.

Tuesday morning, Jack was at my door with two cups of lousy coffee, feeling guilty, feeling like he should be supportive while talking about how this was affecting *him*. I let him drive me to my appointment, but I didn't let him stay. I knew that it hurt him—me pushing him away—but having the wrong kind of support was worse than not having it from him at all. We were early, and Jill met us across the street at a French bakery that had a sign with a little blue Eiffel Tower on it. I picked at layers of a flaky croissant, not eating more than a bite. My fingers felt greasy, and the vague nausea felt less vague and more focused. R.E.M.'s "Night Swimming" was playing softly over the speakers.

Jack gave me an awkward hug in the parking lot in front of the little blue Eiffel Tower sign.

"I feel like I should stay."

"I don't want you to stay."

I left him there, in the middle of the parking lot looking uneasy, and Jill and I walked to the office in a little brick building that looked like an English cottage. Inside, it smelled like a Crabtree & Evelyn store, but with sharp notes of antiseptic soap.

The waiting room was wallpapered, and it made me think about the wallpaper in my childhood bedroom—Laura Ashley, white with tiny blue flowers. It all looked too soft and cheery for how I was feeling. My nose began running. I filled out the forms and Jill squeezed my hand. We waited. The clock on the wall ticked with a vengeance against the silence in the room.

Jill tried to make conversation and talked about some party that we should go to on Friday. Halloween was a week away, and it was a costume party. I wasn't really listening but I nodded in time to the ringing in my ears and the ticking of the angry clock. Even though I wasn't high, everything was still blunted from last night's heroin.

The nurse called me in and took my blood; I went to the bathroom and peed in a cup. The doctor came in and told me what I already knew: "Well, you are pregnant." She explained the procedure and the ringing in my ears got louder. I heard the word *suction* and a wave of nausea passed through me.

Later, on a table, I felt everything above me—light and color and life vanish. I heard the doctor's voice, but I couldn't make out the words. It was all so fuzzy, and I couldn't open my eyes. I didn't want to open them anyway. I thought about the Laura Ashley wallpaper, and I thought about a Cabbage Patch doll I had when I was a kid. My mom ran out and got her for me when I was sick at home. It was a surprise; they were sold out everywhere. The doll's shirt was yellow. I couldn't remember what I called her. I wondered where she was.

Time was unclear; I'd been lying there five minutes or five hours. I heard the words *you're all done.*

The fuzziness of the twilight receded and a new feeling of grief smothered me. I didn't see it coming. Alone in the room, I cried uncontrollably and inconsolably, and I was desperate to shove all these emotions back inside. I craved apathy, distance. I sat up, and a sharp stabbing cramp took my breath. If I narrowed in on the pain, it took the shape and sensation of all the shame I'd ever felt in my body, of my body. I willed myself to push forward. Dressing, I could barely stand up. The nurse came in and told me to lie back down and wait for the twilight to wear off more.

Trapped. *I am trapped in these cramps and this blood and my limbs and shoulders and chest and feet. I am trapped in this room that smells like Crabtree & Evelyn and antiseptic soap. My skin is on fire, and I want to rip it off and escape this pain body.*

Jill drove me home and tucked me in and went to make us tea. The whistle of the kettle sounded an alarm inside me, and I felt what I can only describe as God's judgment. *I don't believe in God.* I felt my judgment. *You're twenty-six and you just killed a baby, your baby; you'll never have a child now.* My mind fought back and reasoned that I didn't want children, reasoned that I've never believed in God, and reasoned that there needs to be a choice, that unwanted children should not be brought into this world. And I hated myself for feeling guilty. *The Cabbage Patch doll's shirt was yellow and I can't remember what I called her.*

Jill brought me the tea and wanted to stay, but I told her I just wanted to sleep. That was a lie. Once she was gone, I drove back to the Valley. I shouldn't have been driving. My skin was on fire, my soul was on fire, and I couldn't see straight. *It wasn't supposed to be like this. I'm pro-choice. I don't want children. This was all a big mistake. I did the right thing.* These thoughts ran through my head in a hamster wheel that spun faster and faster and then my brain was on fire, too.

"You look tired," Juan said as he took $200 out of my hand and passed me a handful of dirty blue balloons.

Jack kept calling. I didn't answer; I turned my phone off.

It was dark when I got home and I was cold; I didn't wear a jacket. The cramps had me doubling over in the elevator. When I got inside the condo, I crawled to the bathroom, in pain, on fire, overwhelmed with mourning for a child I didn't want, I couldn't want. The bathroom floor was cold but did nothing to put out the fire.

I did the only thing I thought would help: I got high.

It took a lot of heroin to get there. I smoked two balloons' worth. It didn't blot out the grief completely, but everything dimmed. I felt myself drifting, drifting again, faster and further. I didn't care; I wanted to fall.

Jack's snoring from the living room woke me up. For the third night that week, he hadn't come to bed, and I was grateful. I didn't want him to touch me. I didn't want to smell him; I could barely look him in the eye. He'd stopped paying close attention to me. And for that, I was grateful, too. From the moment I found out I was pregnant, I felt myself backing away from him, like I was suddenly allergic to all the parts of him that had once attracted me.

I saw my reflection in the dark bathroom mirror. I'd accidentally left the door cracked open. The shadows on my face made me look like a monster, and I remembered that I dreamed of the corpse baby. It had been almost three weeks since the abortion, and I was strung out, again, and hiding it from everyone, including Jack. I felt nothing. That's not true; I felt hatred, for myself.

I grabbed my cell phone to check the time: 9:45 a.m.—not too early to call Juan. He didn't answer. I figured he was still asleep. His girlfriend had thrown him out and he'd been sleeping in a trailer near the railroad tracks in North Hollywood. There was a whole community of people living in these trailers in an industrial park behind some warehouses. I wondered how that was legal. Then I felt guilty.

My stomach cramped. *Thank God, I don't have to work today.* I couldn't bear the thought of painting my face and putting on a dress and making small talk with stylists and celebrity assistants peddling clothes for commercials and photo shoots. When I'd called in, I could tell in CeCe's voice that she knew I wasn't really sick, or at least not the kind of sick I pretended to be.

I called Juan again. No answer, so I peeked in on Jack, passed out, an old cigarette butt in his hand. *Asshole. I told him not to smoke in my apartment.*

I put on a Stones CD and took a shower. "Torn and Frayed" came on and I felt the invisible loaded gun in my invisible pocket. This song always reminded me of Pete. He'd put it on the jukebox at Swingers the first night we hung out, sharing a Burst of Blue shake and some fries. I shut my eyes and let the water pelt my face. Pete—tall, golden-haired, with these beautiful high cheekbones and full lips. His teeth were kind of fucked up, in that European way, which was my favorite part of him. I knew the first time I saw him that I wanted to be with him, not just sleep with him, but be with him. Pete. I fucked that one up. I can spin it any way I like, but I left him because Jack was more exciting, Jack paid attention to me, Jack made me feel sexy. Jack still had some rock star swagger left over, and I fell for him like a cheap trick. I didn't love Jack. I couldn't. That wasn't his fault.

I saw Pete at a Halloween party, a week after the abortion, the party Jill told me about, and I think he knew I was high. No one else did, I'm sure of that, but Pete knew me. He knew every part of me, the darkest parts and maybe the light parts, too. I listened to "Torn and Frayed" over and over in the shower, wishing things had turned out differently.

I called Juan, another ten times. No answer. Jack was still passed out. I used the guest bathroom, which I rarely went into, and saw Jack's compact mirror sitting on the sink. I frequently saw him carry it around with him. I opened it. There was a folded piece of tinfoil with a chunk of tar heroin in it. *Motherfucker.* Although I'd been using for the better part of three weeks, hiding it from him, I was angry. Back in the living room, I pulled his wallet out of his crumpled pants on the floor and looked for more evidence. There it was, two balloons and a tiny plastic bag with what looked like soap shavings. I was fairly sure it was crack because it looked like what that asshole near MacArthur Park tried to sell me a few years ago.

Jack finally woke up. I didn't mention what I found; I left it where it was. I wasn't ready to confront his mess or mine. Instead, I told Jack I was going to run errands and drove to Juan's trailer. When I arrived, I didn't see his truck. Some kids were playing outside and I wondered why they weren't in school. The place smelled like burnt rubber.

Juan's trailer door was ajar and I pushed it open. The trailer was a mess. It smelled like ammonia. Juan's cousin was there. I didn't know his name. He was wearing a turquoise shirt that said I'm Mr. Happy, and he was sweating as he kept touching the thin dark mustache on his upper lip. He barely spoke English and I don't speak Spanish, but I managed to comprehend that Juan got arrested. I asked his cousin if he could get me some "cheeba." He acted like he understood and motioned for me to sit down, but I didn't.

He went to the back of the trailer and came back with a beer and something behind his back. He set the beer down and put his hand on my shoulder and pressed down hard, forcing me to sit on the ground. He started unzipping his pants and motioned for me to get on my knees and suck his dick. I shook my head and said no, dizzy from the smell of ammonia in the cramped trailer.

"You want cheeba? I have Juan cheeba."

For a split second I felt desperate, the invisible loaded gun in my invisible pocket pressed on my leg, and I considered sucking his dick. I thought, *I could just let him rape me. I deserve this.* The corpse baby flashed through my mind. *She's wearing a yellow shirt.*

He brought his arm out from behind his back and showed me a dildo and pulled me forward, so my chin hit the floor of the trailer.

"You like it? You like it?"

I froze as he pulled me up and shoved his hand down the front of my pants and rubbed my cheek with the dildo. He removed his hand, threw the dildo on the couch, and said something in Spanish I didn't understand. He took his dick out and was stroking himself while he turned to get a swig of his beer.

I started feeling back in my body again and an old fury rose inside me. I jumped to my feet, knocking into him, knocking the beer out of his hand.

"Fuck off!"

He grabbed my wrist and I kicked his arm until he let go and I stumbled down the trailer steps. I could hear him behind me and I started to run.

When I got to my car, I looked up. The children outside had stopped playing and stared at me as I got in my car. I drove off, shaky, and pulled over on a residential street a few minutes later to catch my breath. Most of the women I know who've been addicted to heroin were assaulted or raped at least once while scoring drugs. I am profoundly lucky that I got away. If I hadn't, I'd never have reported it. Instead, I'd have added it to the layers of shame I already carried.

On the way home, I called Juan's sometimes girlfriend, Vanessa, to see if she was holding. She filled me in on what had happened. There was a bust at the trailer. Juan and a couple of other guys got arrested but then released, and Juan was on his way back to Mexico. Vanessa didn't have anything but said she might tomorrow. I told her about Juan's cousin.

"Shit. I'm sorry. Juan is gonna be soooo pissed."

By the time I got home, Jack had left, and I was sure he'd gone to buy drugs. I lay down on the couch and tried to ignore my increasing withdrawal symptoms. I was sweaty and cramping and anxious. When Jack got back, I told him we needed to talk.

"Yeah, okay. I just have to piss."

He was in there awhile and I knew what he was doing; I could smell it.

"Open the door."

Silence.

"I know you're getting high."

I could hear him blowing smoke as he said, "I'm just going to the bathroom. Jeez."

Stupidly, he didn't lock the door, and I opened it to find him standing with a piece of tinfoil in one hand and a tinfoil straw in the other. He started to spew excuses that I wasn't interested in hearing. I grabbed the drugs out of his hand and took a big hit. He stood there, mouth agape. *Idiot*, I thought. He had no idea I was using. I told him that I had been. And then I asked him to go get some more.

Jack came back later with more dope and some crack. Crack, like any form of cocaine, never had appealed to me and it represented some line in my addiction I didn't want to cross. I'd seen what crack did to people, how it made a bad situation even worse, how it pushed people to use more heroin and, in turn, more crack. I'd seen people on crack act belligerent and irrational and out of control in ways I'd yet to be. But as the night went on, and he asked me if I wanted some, that invisible loaded gun came out of my invisible pocket, and I put it in my mouth and took my first hit of crack cocaine.

I sent Jack out again for more crack and he came back and I wanted him to fuck me. For the first time since I found out I was pregnant, I wanted him to fuck me, and he couldn't fuck me hard enough, and the corpse baby flashed in my mind, and I thought about Juan's sweaty cousin standing there in his "I'm Mr. Happy" shirt with the dildo and the bottle of beer, and I thought about that doctor's office and the smell of Crabtree & Evelyn, and I thought about the Cabbage Patch doll, and I thought about Pete and his hair and his cheeks and his teeth and his hands, and the corpse baby flashed in my mind, and I asked Jack to choke me and to fuck me harder and he couldn't do it hard enough—*and she had a yellow shirt and I can't remember what I called her*—and I wanted him to hurt me, I wanted him to hurt me so bad that I stopped seeing the corpse baby.

He got tired and couldn't finish and I needed to come down, get low, so I went to the bathroom and smoked some more dope. I turned on "Torn and Frayed" and got in the shower and washed and washed and scratched my arms and legs until I bled.

CHAPTER 16
Whitey
Thanksgiving Day 2000

I pressed my cheek against the cold windowpane and looked with one eye at the horizon, where the gray sky and the gray water of the Sakonnet River met. It was Thanksgiving morning, and Jack and I had flown in the day before to spend the long weekend in Rhode Island at Dad's. We didn't bring enough dope with us; it was almost gone, and my mind kicked into high gear—on a mission to avoid getting dope-sick.

I told Dad we were going to an AA meeting at Providence College, a fact I vetted in the meeting directory. Jack and I set off in search of another kind of recovery. We had no connections in this city and he wanted to find a methadone clinic. I thought that would take too long and instead drove toward the other side of the I-95, the side that holds the projects, wanting to try our luck there.

There was barely anyone out; I noticed the police station was across the street from the projects. I didn't care. We pulled over next to a mini market that was in what looked like a small white shed. Jack got out and asked some guy, in his "black voice," if he knew where we could get some horse. The guy didn't even answer, so Jack got back in the car.

"You know, it's insulting that you talk to black guys in your 'black voice,'" I said.

"Oh, shut up."

"It's true. It's not just insulting, it's racist."

He looked annoyed and lit a cigarette. I reminded him he couldn't smoke in the car and he got out, walked down the street. I looked across at the rows of identical brick buildings and watched as two kids raced across the barren yard. I felt myself sinking with another type of shame, one that went beyond my desperation for heroin. *I make myself sick.*

I'd felt shame about my socioeconomic privilege for as long as I'd been aware of it, since I was in elementary school. At lunch, a girl called me a rich bitch because I'd casually said I only wore Guess jeans while we ate our sandwiches. I remember the heat rising in my cheeks. The girl lived in a small apartment near the school with her mom and didn't come to school wearing brand-name anything. It had never occurred to me that what I said would make someone else feel badly.

The more my father gave me, the more extravagant the gift, the worse I felt, yet I couldn't extricate myself from the pull of monetary affection. I felt guilty that I had everything I had and still wanted to die. As an adult, as a heroin addict, it was impossible to ignore the communities I ventured into to buy drugs. I felt culpable for being part of the ecosystem that kept people in poverty, especially people of color. But the need for heroin was stronger than anything my conscience could argue.

I looked in my rearview mirror and saw a big black guy approaching, and watched him go into the little market. I got out of the car and waited for him to return. When he did, I spoke to him—*in my regular voice.*

"Hey."

He looked me up and down, like he was trying to work out what I wanted, and said, "Hey, what you need?"

"Heroin," I said.

"It's your lucky day. What's your name?"

"Erin."

"Erin. I'm Whitey. Stay here."

When Jack returned, I was waiting, leaning against the car, $300 ready inside my glove.

"I'm cold, I'm pissed, and I feel like shit. Let's go drive around some more. We should have gone to find a methadone clinic like I said to begin with," he said.

"Just get back in the car. Whitey's coming back."

"Whitey?"

"Just get in the car. I've got this."

Whitey came back, and I noticed just how tall he was. He had to be at least six-five or six-six. I bought ten baggies of powdered heroin and $100 of crack. Whitey took the money I handed him from my glove. He also gave me his cell phone number. Jack hopped out of the car and introduced himself to Whitey, using his "black voice."

Whitey laughed and looked at me and said, "See you soon, Erin."

We made it back to Dad's and his girlfriend, Stacy, was there, cooking. Stacy had just adopted a little girl named Anya from Russia. She was still a baby really, two years old. Anya's face was big and round and pale like a doll. She was sweet but hesitant— unsure about receiving the love and affection everyone was wrapping around her like tinsel. Her big blue eyes were watery, and I was sure she saw my corpse baby dancing in my pupils when she looked at me. She wanted to sit with me, have me read to her, and I felt like I shouldn't even touch her. I didn't want to smear my sadness on her face.

During dinner, Anya sat on Dad's lap and called him Da-da. I didn't remember ever sitting on my dad's lap, but surely I did.

I must have at one time, right? Part of me was jealous of Anya, jealous of the way she sat comfortably in his lap. I wanted to be two again and be held by my father, even if I couldn't remember that he ever had. Later, I told him that he should marry Stacy and be Anya's da-da or let them go and stop playing father to a baby girl who had none.

"Are you all right?" Dad asked me. "You don't look well."

"Me? Yeah, I'm good."

He looked intently at me, and I knew he didn't believe me.

"You know, I was thinking—well, more than thinking, kind of planning—that I want to go back to school and graduate."

"Back to USC? I think that's a good idea."

"Yeah. I already called, and I can start back in January. Is that okay? Will you help me with the tuition?"

"Okay," he said.

On the face of things, the conversation was normal, cordial, but I knew from his body language and the way he looked at me that he was onto me; he knew.

Later, after everyone else had gone to sleep, Jack and I went down to the basement and watched *The Perfect Storm*. The movie upset me for some reason, and I kept going to the bathroom to smoke crack and blow it out the window. The cold air from outside felt so fucking cold and my mind started to race. I thought about Anya upstairs asleep—innocent and deserving of all the love. Thinking about Anya led me to thinking about my corpse baby, and the dreams I'd been having where I would see the baby's face, perfect in every way except blue and bloody. I hated myself for not being able to have the abortion and move on with my life. I hated myself for not being able to disconnect from my womb and what it made me feel. I hated myself for making an abortion a fully developed corpse baby that followed me wherever I went.

Late that night or early the next morning, I slept a little and dreamed about a wave, like the one in *The Perfect Storm*—

a wave so big that it obliterated everything in its path. I was stuck in the wave, and it didn't kill me, but it didn't let me go either. Then I saw that Anya was in the wave. I couldn't save her, and she was dead—underwater, floating like my corpse baby, and she was wearing a yellow shirt, and I couldn't remember her name.

On Friday, Stacy's ex-husband dropped off their thirteen-year-old daughter, Laura, with her friend. We all headed to Providence to go Black Friday shopping. We took separate cars, and I stopped to get gas so Jack and I could break off from the mini caravan and do our own shopping with Whitey. Jack and I met Whitey at the market again, and we bought more crack and more heroin. After meeting up with everyone and spending time at the mall—pretending to shop and snorting heroin in the bathroom of Nordstrom—we went out for my birthday dinner at my favorite Italian restaurant. It was the one near the loft that had almost been my home with Pete.

It had been my actual birthday the week before. I turned twenty-seven, and all day long I thought, *Twenty-seven is a good age to die.* I met Pete for lunch, which I didn't mention to Jack. In the months since our breakup, Pete had worked to maintain a friendship with me. I wanted one, too, but when we saw each other, I always wanted more and that want left me feeling raw inside.

He was working on the Warner Brothers lot and I met him at Bob's Big Boy in Toluca Lake. I picked at my fries and burger, really only wanting the chocolate shake, while Pete asked me questions that I tried to avoid. By the end of lunch, I admitted I was using, which he already knew. Pete promised to keep my secret safe and told me that he could help me, that he would be there for me. I wanted to tell him that the problem was bigger than drugs. I wanted to tell him I was even more broken than when we were together, that part of me had died with the corpse baby, whose presence I now felt constantly. But letting him think it was just the drugs, that it wasn't some deep-seated dysfunction was more bearable. I didn't want him to know how far gone I was again.

On Saturday, Laura wanted to go to the Christmas tree farm. Laura was tall for her age and, like her mom, had a wholesome face with dimples and an all-American quality that I knew my dad loved. She was everything I wasn't. I was darker; I was too *other*. Everyone went, even Jack, on the tree hunt except me. I took my dad's car and drove back to Providence to meet Whitey. There were a lot of people out.

Whitey got in the car with me, and we went for a drive because he was worried about the cops. I was worried about the time and beating everyone back to the house to avoid any suspicion.

When I pulled up to Dad's house, I could see they were already back. I turned the car around and ran to the grocery store to buy a couple of magazines and some ice cream—proof of where I was. They seemed to buy it, but later Jack told me my dad asked him if I was using again. Of course, Jack denied it.

Sunday afternoon, just before the car picked us up for the airport, Dad pulled me aside and asked, "Are you taking drugs again?"

"No way. Why would you even say that?"

I was impressed that he caught on so quickly this time, he never had before, but I was indignant with my denial. At the airport, I caught a glimpse of myself in the mirrored corridor, in my long Marni hippie dress, knee-high boots, and vintage faux fur. I looked like shit. I looked like a weird, sad clown. I looked like a crazy burned-out hippie. I looked like a junkie.

We boarded the plane. *Twenty-seven is a good age to die.* The confinement of the airplane pressurized the contents of my brain. I wanted to get out, but since I couldn't, I went to the bathroom and smoked crack. I came back to my seat and searched the faces of everyone around me for signs. *Do they know what I was doing? Did I set the smoke alarm off? Can they smell the crack?* The paranoia became intolerable; I returned to the bathroom and snorted some heroin and came back to my seat.

"Jack," I whispered, shaking his arm. "Wake up. Wake up."

"What?"

"Wake up."

Jack groaned, "Come on, what is it?"

"When we get home, I want you to fuck me."

He mumbled and went back into his nod. I repeated this series of actions over and over for the duration of the flight. Jack slept through most of it, save the moments I woke him to tell him I wanted him to fuck me later. By this point in our relationship, I was no longer attracted to him but I wanted him to be part of the dark, chemical wave—a wave strong enough to blot out everything because what I was doing wasn't enough. The heroin and crack weren't giving me the release I needed. They couldn't fix me; I was too broken.

By the time we made our initial descent into LAX, I was certain the flight attendants knew what I'd been doing, especially that bitchy blonde one who smiled at everyone but me. I woke Jack up again.

"They're going to arrest me. Do something," I whispered.

"What are you talking about? Calm down."

"They know, they know. Or at least the blonde one knows."

"Know what?"

"That I've been smoking crack. I think I set off the smoke alarm."

"Why the fuck did you do that?"

I didn't reply. I sat in silence, sweating, fearful tears streaming down my cheeks. I stopped breathing and wondered if I was having a heart attack. The blonde attendant whispered to the older brunette one.

Is she pointing at me? This is it. This is that moment. Twenty-seven is a good age to die. It's not a good age to go to jail.

The wheels touched down, I was soaking with sweat, and I had my hand on the seat belt like the trigger of a gun. I didn't dare unbuckle it before the seat belt light went off. When it did, I grabbed my coat and my bag, and I squeezed myself into the aisle, in the line of passengers. Just another regular flyer here, not one who spent the whole flight in and out of the bathroom committing felonies. As I exited the plane, I looked around the terminal for my arresting officers.

Maybe I'm in the clear, or maybe they're still walking over, maybe the blonde flight attendant, or the older brunette one she tattled to, is calling security right now, or calling the police right now, maybe my arresting officers are waiting for me at baggage claim.

I waited for Jack to catch up with me and told him he had to get the bags. I waited outside and smoked a cigarette, the mild LA air cooling my sweat. I kept looking over my shoulder, suspicious of the sea of faces of people trying to get home after Thanksgiving.

When we got to my apartment, I no longer wanted Jack to fuck me; he looked tired anyway. I gave him a little bit of the dope, and he took his place on the couch, watching *Cops* and nodding out. I took the last of Whitey's crack and went up to the roof of my building and smoked it, in the one corner where I knew the security cameras couldn't see me. I walked to the ledge and looked out at Hollywood below me. A siren droned on. *Twenty-seven is a good age to die.* I believed that. I wish I could wrap that twenty-seven-year-old girl in my arms and tell her that she has so much life in front of her, life that won't be consumed by wanting to die. But the me then wouldn't have believed it.

I found one last crack rock and Whitey's phone number on a piece of a cigarette carton. I climbed up on the ledge and sat and let my feet sway. I closed my eyes and saw the dark wave.

It didn't kill me but it didn't let me go. I saw my corpse baby, floating, blue and bloody and still, and with sadness etched on its cherubic face. Inching toward the edge, I wanted the wave to kill me or to let me go. *Tomorrow, maybe tomorrow, maybe tomorrow.*

CHAPTER 17

Resolutions

January 2001

On New Year's Day 2001, I lay prone on the bedroom floor, covering my face with the long, sheer, blue-and-purple curtain made of sari fabric, which I never hung up properly. The curtain smelled like cigarettes. I propped my feet up on the windowsill. My stomach churned, and I surveyed the damage of the past month.

In December, I quit my job at the boutique and reenrolled at USC. In my last couple of weeks at work, CeCe asked me, more than once, if I was using. I adamantly said no and stopped speaking to her.

I went to Lila's graduation party at her mom's house; she'd finished law school. Jack and I arrived late and high; we smoked crack in the car outside. Lila pulled me aside and asked me if I was okay. "Of course!" I said, and then I stopped speaking to her.

Christmas was a disaster. I spent it dope-sick on my uncle's couch. I told my mom I had the flu. The day after Christmas, Jack and I flew back to Rhode Island to be with my dad—a terrible idea. The first day there, I couldn't get in touch with

Whitey. By day two, we were out of dope and went looking for him. I met a twelve-year-old named Christopher at the little market next to the projects in Providence. I asked him if he knew where I could find Whitey. It turned out he was Whitey's nephew. It turned out Whitey was shot and killed on Christmas Eve. It turned out Christopher knew what I was looking for. It turned out that I bought drugs from a twelve-year-old. It turned out I bought from him four times that week.

You can always sink lower. It's a good thing I'm not becoming a mother. It turns out I'm worse than I thought.

The drugs were not strong enough to erase the facts. I bought drugs from a little boy. A little boy doesn't start dealing drugs because it's what little boys do. A little boy starts dealing drugs because he is taught, he is shown, that it's inevitable for boys like him to deal. I taught him that—*people like me.* I was part of the overriding problems that keep little black boys, like Christopher, stuck in a cycle of systemic poverty and subjugation. I have thought about Christopher many, many times over the years. I hope he got out. God, I hope he got out. After my own recovery, I've volunteered my time and energy and resources in ways that work to end these cycles.

It's not enough. I know that. I wish I could find him. I wish I could go back and yank him out of that place, stop him from ruining his life with people like me, people like the girl I was. *Christopher, I am sorry.*

My dad confronted me again during this visit. I had asked him for cash, told him that my ATM card was not working. He paused and looked at me for a long time.

"Are you on drugs?" he asked.

"No."

"You promise me you are not taking any drugs?"

"I swear, Dad. I am not on drugs. I haven't. I swear on my life."

He handed me $300.

Jack and I flew back to LA, but this time I didn't smoke any crack on the plane. But I was unraveling. I was no longer existing in the real world in any meaningful way. I started to believe that I was hopeless. I couldn't imagine a life for me that didn't end by overdose or suicide, and, increasingly, those two options seemed like my only way out.

Back home, Jack was on the couch asleep, and I kicked his dangling arm. He woke up momentarily, but I said nothing. I didn't want to wake him up; I just wanted to kick him. I walked to Rock 'n' Roll Ralphs on Sunset, underdressed and freezing.

It was so bright in Ralphs, my eyes throbbed. I bought some Jell-O and some Cool Whip. I had no desire to eat anymore, but I wanted this. They had sweatshirts in Ralphs, football team sweatshirts for the Rose Bowl in a cardboard bin near the bread aisle. I put on a purple Huskies sweatshirt and tore off the tag. As I stood in line, waiting to buy the Jell-O and the Cool Whip and the sweatshirt, a man spoke to me. He repeated himself three times before I registered what he said.

"I said, Huskies fan, eh?"

"Who are the Huskies?" I replied.

There was nothing left to say. I walked home and threw the sweatshirt in the trash chute.

Two weeks later

"Now that I've met you, would you object to never seeing me again?"

The words of the character Claudia in *Magnolia* made something inside me stir and sting and blister. A year ago, I'd watched this film with Pete. We got an Academy screener from a friend. We watched it on a damp Wednesday night, in the days leading up to when I broke down and jabbed myself with a box cutter.

Now I was sitting next to Jack, feeling just as unstable but too high to do anything about it, watching the same movie, relating to the same character, and sweaty with the reminder that I was only moments away from everyone seeing what a monster I'd become. With each relapse, hiding became harder both physically and emotionally. I was carrying more shame than I knew how to handle, and it grew with each relapse, each lie, each hit of crack, each thought I had about the abortion and the corpse baby and Christopher. Another damp Wednesday night in January, another year gone by. I took another hit of crack. School was starting the next week, and I should probably have kicked the drugs then, rather than later. But I didn't know how to stop anything anymore. Right after New Year's, my dad cut me off, something he had never done before, and so I acquainted myself with the pawnshop.

I'd been in a pawnshop before, with Pete, when he was struggling with a different addiction, itching to go to the track. Now I'd become a regular at the one on the corner of Robertson and Wilshire—the nice one, where I'd been with Pete, where I felt less like a junkie and more like a socialite who'd fallen on hard times. And then I became familiar with the one on Melrose and Cahuenga—a family-run place that would take the cheaper stuff the other place wouldn't, where I knew they knew what was wrong with me, but they still managed to treat me with relative kindness.

When I didn't feel up to going, I'd send Jack to Wasteland armed with bags of designer clothing, selling them for next to nothing, just to stay well. More precisely, to stay *not sick*.

Jack got a call from his lawyer; a big royalty check was coming in. If he hadn't got that call, I would have kicked him out. I could barely stand the sight of him. He'd become a symbol for the growing black hole inside me, the black hole filled with heartbreak over Pete and the abortion and the relapse and Jack's general lack of awareness of just how strung out I now was. The biggest difference between me and Jack was that he was a drug addict and I was a mentally ill person pretending that drugs were the problem. Most of the time, I convinced myself this was not true, but increasingly, all I could think about was the invisible gun or the ledge on the roof of my building or the box cutter that could do more to my wrists than it did to my leg. I couldn't recognize the blurred lines between the drugs and my depression and the trauma from sexual abuse. All those things melted together and became the filter through which I saw myself: the monster.

I looked at Jack and he smiled and continued watching the movie. I turned away and thought about Pete. My bones ached with missing him. I should never have broken up with Pete. But I did and I was here with Jack. I couldn't remember it being a choice. It seemed like Jack happened to me.

Perhaps that's how my young adult life unraveled. Things would happen and I pretended I didn't play a part in them. I took steps and pretended I was sitting still. Or maybe I was running wildly, without direction, toward the first wall I could find.

The part in *Magnolia* came on when the characters all start singing along to Aimee Mann's "Wise Up." They sang in unison: "It's not going to stop, until you wise up. It's not going to stop, so just give up." The message was for me. I was ready to give up. Then my phone rang. It was my mother.

"Hello?"

"Hi, honey. What are you up to?"

"Just watching a movie."

"You sound funny."

"I'm just tired."

"Well, your dad called, and he's really worried about you, and he's got me worried about you, too."

"Mom, I'm fine."

"We want you to go back to therapy. I found someone in Pasadena."

I agreed to go because it was easier than staying on the phone. *How many therapists and psychiatrists have I been to?* I thought about last January after the leg incident, when Pete and my friend Sunny were looking into mental health care facilities for me.

I thought about that afternoon when I sat with my mom and the psychiatrist. *We don't really know if that happened.* I thought about the therapist Pete and I had gone to, Karen, and how she helped me and how I missed her. I thought about Dr. Gregory and my anger and being fourteen and four and eight and twenty-one, and *twenty-seven is a good age to die.*

Jack was asleep, and the final scene in *Magnolia* played, and Claudia had hope finally, and Aimee Mann sang "Save Me," and I wondered if I would ever feel hopeful again. I wondered if I was too far gone. I wondered if I would ever forgive myself for having an abortion. I wondered if I would ever get over Pete. I wondered if the monster I saw in the mirror would ever go away.

I wondered if I could *want* to live again.

CHAPTER 18
Sympathy for the Roach
February 2001

"It's nice to meet you, Erin."

"Nice to meet you, too, Joanne."

"Just call me Jo. So, tell me why you're here today?"

I smiled at the therapist. Just-Call-Me-Jo. And blinked, noticing how dry my eyes were.

"Well, I'm here because my mother is concerned that I've been depressed, I guess."

"So, tell me, are you depressed?"

"Define *depressed*. I'm not not-depressed."

"So, tell me how you define depression?"

"I guess I'm not happy. I mean it's been a rough year. Um, how do I define depression? I guess it's a vacuum. It just sucks everything away, good and bad. It's not really sadness. It's like inertia."

"So, tell me, do you feel that's where you are now, in a vacuum?"

"No. Maybe."

"Your mother expressed concern to me that you may be using drugs again. So, tell me, do you think drugs are part of what's going on with you?"

I wanted to tell Just-Call-Me-Jo to shove her *so, tell me*s up her ass. I also wanted to tell her that the Santa Fe color scheme in her office was making me nauseous. Instead, I said, "I'm not using."

"So, tell me then, why do you think your mother is concerned?"

I told Just-Call-Me-Jo that I had an abortion and that it was unexpectedly devastating and that I didn't tell anyone and that I resented Jack and that I was not on drugs, but I was just sad about the abortion. Some of this was true. She suggested that I open up to my mother, and she suggested that I come back on Monday, and she suggested that talk therapy could be the answer.

I didn't tell her about the leg incident or the PTSD. I didn't tell her about the heroin or the crack or how I fucked things up with Pete or the corpse baby or the invisible gun in my invisible pocket or how I fantasized about getting really high and letting myself float right off the roof of my building. I took her card with my appointment time for Monday and drove to Mom's like I promised her I would.

I pulled up in front of my mom and stepdad's home, an English traditional on a leafy street in South Pasadena that looked cozy against the dark gray sky that threatened to rain at any moment. My relationship with my mother had been muddled by the sting of her words the year before in the psychiatrist's office. We had yet to talk any more about the sexual abuse, and at the time, I didn't understand how painful it was for her to confront. I couldn't see past my own wounds. But my mom *was* trying to be there, wanted to be there, and that did count for something; it counted for a lot.

My mom made me a cup of tea, and we sat at the island in her kitchen.

"How did it go?" she asked.

"It was good. I feel better."

"Oh, good! Are you going to see her again?"

"Yeah, I made another appointment for Monday."

"I'm glad, honey."

I clinked the spoon around in my cup and said, "Mom, I kind of need to tell you something."

As the words came out of my mouth, I hadn't decided what exactly I was going to tell her.

"What is it, honey?"

"I know you or Dad think that I've been using. But that's not it. I have been keeping something from you, though." *I can't believe I am about to deflect with this.* "I had an abortion in October."

My tears came immediately. I didn't know if I was crying about the abortion or the corpse baby or the lies I was still telling. She cried, too, and hugged me and told me she knew I wasn't on drugs, that something else was going on. Then she pulled back and looked at me.

"I want you to swear to me you're not using."

I looked at her watery face and her watery gray-green eyes and said, "Mom, I swear, I'm not using."

She hugged me again, and I could feel her tears on my neck. I knew she loved me. I thought again of the psychiatrist's office the year before. *We don't know if that really happened.* How could she know? I hardly gave her the chance to know anything about me.

I wanted to stay there in my mom's embrace forever. I wanted to go back to being a little girl when she brought me warm clothes out of the dryer on cold mornings; when she cut up slices of apples and cheese for me at night; when she sang "Chantilly Lace" and we burst into giggles at the line "make me feel real loose, like a long-necked goose;" when she called me Childie McBride—a nickname I never understood but loved. I wanted to go back to those small moments in which I felt safe and protected. For one brief second while I hugged my mom, all the tension in my bones and jaw and skin released. I forgave her, for everything. And then just as quickly as the release, the addiction inside me pulled everything taut again.

I excused myself and called Jack from the bathroom. His check wasn't going to be in until the next day, and I realized we had no dope and no money for dope and it was getting late.

My mom's phone rang. I could hear her talking in the kitchen; she was on a work call. I sneaked into my mom's room and sat down on the edge of her bed. I moved to her dressing room and looked at the framed poem on the vanity.

I felt
Sympathy
For the roach
I squashed
Against the wall,
Who in his little
Mind
Had thought
The world
His own.

I can't say how many times I had recited those lines in my head. My mother cut this poem, titled "Unwary," out of a newspaper when she was a child and kept it as an adult, in a special black lacquered box on her dresser. I used to sneak into my parents' room, open the box, and remove the clipping. Now she kept it in a frame on her vanity.

My earliest memories of the poem are from when I was three years old and my grandfather, my mother's father, was diagnosed with lung cancer. My mom came home on a warm September afternoon, and I sensed a shift within her that scared me—a shift that signified things I had yet to understand.

At that age, I idolized my mom and hated that we didn't look alike. Although I was a pretty child, I never liked my appearance. My hair was straight and brown, with matching brown eyes. My olive skin seemed greenish next to her golden Swedish complexion. My reflection was murky and hers glowed. She was all warmth and beauty in my mind. Tall and slender with long, wavy flaxen hair and green eyes that seemed to smile even through sadness. She turned heads when she entered a room. That warm September afternoon, her green eyes turned gray and her posture stiffened.

Grandpa's cancer was swift and unrelenting. By Christmas, he was in the midst of chemo, vomiting blood and visibly wasting away. That shift in my mom—that I had felt three months earlier—swelled and I saw her wasting away alongside her father. I was no longer welcome in my parents' bed at night. Instead, I sat silently in my dark bedroom, listening to my mother's sobbing from down the hall.

The sound of her crying triggered insomnia that would stay with me into adulthood. It was worse when I didn't hear her crying. My heart would pound, and I would sit against my door, ear pressed firmly, in an attempt to decipher the silence. My mind wandered erratically in the quiet times, trying to escape the ache I had for the warm and happy mother who no longer existed.

In early March, at four years old, I was at my preschool climbing on the cold steel train in the yard. It was a wet, cool afternoon. I stretched back on the train and let my head dangle upside down, watching parents retrieve their children. My grandfather had been in the hospital since early January and my mom was often late picking me up. But watching the clouds loom above, a strange new sensation spread through me. Panic. I struggled to remember if my mom had ever been this late. The blood rushing to my head, I began to feel dizzy. I let the wooziness wash over me and shut my eyes, trying to quiet this feeling of dread.

Through the gate, I saw my mother's best friend, Olga. I sat up straight and took a loud breath. The damp air felt soft on my cheeks. We got in her car and she explained that my parents were at the hospital. We headed to McDonald's; I was thrilled. Mom never took me to McDonald's. The heat in the car spread from my toes, up my legs, and I noticed a scrape on my knee.

Enjoying my Happy Meal, I stared through the window at the large raindrops beating down on the cars outside. They were loud and got louder still. Olga spoke.

"Erin-ie. I have to tell you something. Your grandpa died this morning. I'm so sorry, troll."

Olga's pet name for me was troll, and her Swedish accent calmed me. I wasn't sure how I felt or how I was supposed to feel. Worried about my mom, my scraped knee began to throb and I felt trapped by the stuffiness of the room and my coat. I said nothing and continued to eat my salty fries and pick at the sugary hamburger bun. The food pushed down the lump in my throat.

That evening, my father picked me up from Ken and Olga's and told me that my mom was home, sleeping. He sang, off-key, to the Linda Ronstadt song on the radio.

"I'm going back someday, come what may, to Blue Bayou…"

In the back seat of my father's car, I stared out the window into the black sky, the clouds obscuring any hope of seeing a star. The lump in my throat began to rise, and I strained to push it back down with thoughts of Blue Bayou. *Where was Blue Bayou? Was it a real place?* It sounded magnificent and I focused on it, keeping my shaky emotions locked away.

I did not see my mom that night, nor did I see her the next day, or the day after that. She slept and slept and slept. I wondered if maybe she was dying, too. Every morning before she was up, I was whisked out of the house. My afternoons were spent at Olga and Ken's, playing with their daughter Sara, who was like a sister to me, our parents close like siblings. I was okay during the day. But at night, after my father had picked me up and driven me home, the panic I had just learned to feel mounted with each of the twenty-eight steps that led to our front door.

My grandpa's funeral was held a few days after he died. I was not allowed to attend. But I did finally see my mom that morning. I knocked on the bedroom door and she whispered, "Come in."

Like an apparition, she sat at her vanity, so withdrawn she nearly wasn't there. She looked thin and breakable. Her wavy hair was dull and limp and her smiling gray-green eyes sank deeply into her face. I searched her features for something more familiar, something comforting, but I couldn't find what I was looking for, so I ran to her and threw my arms around her waist.

"I love you, Mommy. I'm sorry about Grandpa."

She responded by clutching me too tightly and weeping. After a few minutes, she let go and proceeded to get ready. I sat on the bed watching her, noticing how she seemed different and worrying she would stay this way forever. As she was rummaging through her closet, she screamed. I jumped to my feet and ran to her.

"What, Mommy? What's wrong? What's wrong?"

Moths flew out of her closet.

"God damn it! God damn it!" she yelled, yanking her clothes down and throwing them across the room.

She sat on the floor, put her head in her hands, and bawled. I waited for things to quiet. Placing my hand on her head, I offered the only advice I could muster with my four years of experience.

"Mommy, one day, you'll look back on this and laugh."

I'm sure I had heard that somewhere before.

She did laugh, at first, until the laughter became tears and she turned away from me.

I ran to my room and buried my head in Henry, a six-foot-tall yellow stuffed dog that my uncle bought for me after a big win in Las Vegas. I felt like I should cry, but I didn't. Instead, I lay there in Henry's lap and counted how many seconds I could hold my breath.

I heard the babysitter arrive and my parents leave. Thankfully, the sitter left me alone. I tiptoed down the hallway into my parents' room and opened the special black lacquered box on my mom's dresser. Slowly, I pulled out its treasures. I held her baby teeth in my hands and saw that my grandfather's watch and rings were in the box, too. I opened her bottle of perfume—Opium—and dabbed some on my wrists and behind my ears like I had seen her do. Then I took out the newspaper clipping and lay down on the bed. Holding the paper just above my head, I put my new reading skills to work.

"I felt sympathy for the roach I squashed against the wall, who in his little mind had thought the world his own."

Something stirred. I was struck by an overwhelming sense of loneliness. I read the words out loud, three or four times, and the tears finally came. I cried for the first time since my grandpa died. I cried for the roach, for losing my grandpa, for my mother's sadness, and for the divestiture of the mother I had before—the mother who was all warmth and beauty and who kept me safe. That mother was gone, and in her place, I was left with a ghost. Behind the sadness and loneliness, I felt terrified. Sadness was a wave. It could steal people. It could leave you with nothing.

Turning my head to the side, I placed my wrist over my mouth and nose and inhaled, losing myself in her scent.

Now, twenty-three years later, I sat at her vanity and looked around for a bottle of Opium, not finding one. I took a handful of items—a couple of rings and pendants—out of a jewelry drawer. I stuck them in my pocket, and I felt hot and guilty and nauseous. Back in the kitchen, my mom was still on the phone. I hugged her goodbye and left my tears on her sweater. I whispered, *"I'm sorry. I forgive you."* She didn't hear me. Maybe I didn't say it out loud.

On the way home, I stopped at the pawnshop on Cahuenga and Melrose. It was crowded and I had to wait. The rain outside was relentless and everyone inside smelled like wet dirt and body odor. I got a $100 loan on two rings and called my new dealer, Gaela. I was anxious to meet up; I hadn't fixed since that morning before therapy.

I got to our spot. And I waited. And I waited. I'd spent an eternity there, waiting for Gaela. I know I'm exaggerating, but that hardly matters. There, in the parking lot of Burger King, on the corner of Third Street and Alvarado, I waited and I waited. She was thirty minutes late and I was dope-sick.

At thirty-five minutes and counting, I headed into Burger King. The smell inside made me even more nauseous: bleach, dirty mop, french fries, beef, and an overriding metallic odor, like blood. I pulled on the bathroom door, realizing it was locked and I didn't have a token. I got in line, ordered a Dr. Pepper, got a token, and made it to the bathroom just in time. My throat and my nostrils burned and I began to dry heave; I could smell the withdrawal in my sweat. I pulled myself together as quickly as possible, splashing cold water on my face, leaving my Dr. Pepper on the sink, panicked at the thought that I might have missed Gaela.

She had been my new dealer since Juan went to jail and his girlfriend stopped dealing. Jack had found Gaela and now it seemed I wasted half my day, every day, waiting for her. I saw Gaela in my side mirror.

Actually, I didn't see Gaela, but I saw her hair approaching. It was a peroxide blond that glowed no matter the time of day or the weather. That helmet of yellow framed her round brown face and her black penciled-in eyebrows. I thought she was Mexican or maybe Guatemalan. I felt like an asshole for not knowing.

She was alone that day. Sometimes she had her baby with her, in a stroller. I wasn't sure if it was a boy or girl, but the presence of that baby always pinched at me. That baby was another reminder of the many lives affected by my drug use, affected by people like me. And the baby reminded me of the corpse baby, confirming yet again how right it was that I not be a mother.

I unlocked my car and she got in the passenger seat.

"Hey," she said.

This was one of the few words Gaela ever said to me in English. Her repertoire could be distilled to *okay, no, hey, bye, twenty minutes, later, yes, call me later,* and *no credit.* Invariably, Gaela got in my car and we'd drive in a big loop, up to Beverly, over to Burlington, back down Third Street, and to her apartment building, right there on Alvarado, like I was just a pal dropping her off at home. The transaction, the exchange of money for drugs, took place on this drive, all done well before we'd reached her place. When the baby was with her, she would fold the stroller, throw it in my trunk, and sit in the back with the baby. Having no car seat, I worried we'd get pulled over.

I dropped her off and my heart raced. My body was weak and eager to get well again. I went back to Burger King, stood in line, ordered a chocolate—peanut butter pie, and got another token. The bathroom smelled like other people's urine and the dry heaving started again. I noticed some piss on the toilet seat and my hands shook. The dope smelled more vinegary than usual and I threw a sticky piece on the foil. *Inhale, it's off, something's not right.* It tasted like shit, shit and vinegar. I hated Gaela and her crappy dope. I took a few more hits and stopped because someone was pounding on the door.

"Just a minute." My voice cracked.

I ran the water for a minute while the vinegar cloud dissipated and opened the door to a man in a motorized wheelchair. He gave me a dirty look. I realized I left the chocolate—peanut butter pie on the sink.

Driving back down Third, heading west, I felt better but sick in a new way, sick from whatever the dope was cut with. I

cursed out Gaela in my mind. The stop-and-go traffic amplified my nausea.

Finally, back home, Jack was there. He was in a good mood
and he had dope. He was able to get his check after all, and
now we had $10,000 and better dope. So I stashed Gaela's crap
heroin away, just in case I needed it for another day, and we got
high—separately, together, all weekend.

Monday morning I got high enough to deal with Just-Call-
Me-Jo but not so high that she noticed.

"So, tell me, did you talk to your mom after our last session?" she asked.

"Yes."

"So, tell me, how did that go?"

"Really, really well."

Liar. Again, it was only part of the truth. I was just loaded
enough that I could pretend I didn't care.

CHAPTER 19

I See You

Valentine's Day 2001

Her mother just looks at her for a long minute, then removes a jade pendant from around her neck and hands it to her daughter. "June, since your baby time, I wear this next to my heart. Now you wear next to yours. It will help you know: I see you. I see you."

—Amy Tan, *The Joy Luck Club*

My mom and I both read *The Joy Luck Club* when I was seventeen and saw the movie together a few years later. The stories reveal the intricate relationships between mothers and daughters. There was one scene that resonated with us both—one of the mothers finally tells her daughter, "I see you." Through unspoken words, we understood how this reflected our relationship, or more accurately the hope we had for our relationship. Like the mother in the book, my mother had a jade pendant. It had belonged to her mother. But she didn't give it to me. Now it was in the pawnshop. She didn't know it was missing.

What my mom did give me for my twenty-first birthday was a white gold Tiffany ID bracelet that was engraved. It read, "I see you." She welled up with tears when she gave it to me and hugged me tighter than she had in years. I loved it but could never bring myself to wear it. I knew she couldn't see me.

She couldn't see the junkie—the one who lied and stole and let boys touch her. She couldn't see the one who got high in the bathrooms of homes and Burger Kings and doctors' offices and gas stations and cars and delis and universities and garages and airports and department store fitting rooms. She couldn't see the one who sat on her hands, holding her breath and counting the seconds when all she wanted to do was grab the box cutter and carve away until the crazy left her body in tiny particles. She couldn't see the one smoking crack in an airplane bathroom and hallucinating the corpse baby she'd aborted. She couldn't see the real me because if she did, she wouldn't love me because nobody can love a monster.

I sat in my car and held the bracelet my mom had given me six years before in the palm of my hand, tracing over the engraving with my finger. I dropped it in the cup holder, grabbed the small bag on the passenger seat, and got out of the car.

Halfway to the apartment door, I turned around to retrieve it. Taking a moment in the car, I lit up a cigarette. Jack was back at the apartment, deep in a nod. The thought of him there annoyed me. Every time I thought of him, my mind went through a list of everything about him that I couldn't stand. We were both in a race, only we were racing toward different things. He was racing toward a high; I was racing toward a low.

My stomach rumbled, and I couldn't remember the last time I ate. Monday? I struggled to recall what day of the week it was and remembered it was Valentine's Day. I didn't fucking care about hearts or chocolate or love. My self-loathing had grown. I could taste it in my mouth, rising from my gut like bile. Self-hatred has a taste all its own. It's bitter and acidic and hard to choke down.

The low I'd been chasing felt lower than ever before. The lower I got, the more I craved getting lower. I wanted to abandon all my senses and remember nothing. I wanted to get so low that I'd forget my name and my body. I no longer wanted to exist.

I read an article years ago about gambling addiction that said that gamblers were chasing a loss, not a win, that they couldn't stop until they lost everything. When I read it, I got hot and dizzy with recognition because that was how I felt, like I couldn't stop going lower, losing more, stripping myself down to nothing. When you believe that you're a monster, fueled by shame, the low can be all that you see. There is no high or anything else left to chase.

I took a drag off my Parliament cigarette and blew smoke out the window, feeling my chest rattle. I'd been smoking more and more crack, and that rattle in my chest had been getting a little worse each day. It was raining, soft at first, and then persistently. The driver's side window of my Volvo was stuck open, and my arm was wet. I felt damp inside, like a thing tossed down the basement stairs—forgotten, musty, broken. A chill coursed through me, straight to my bones.

Leading up to Valentine's Day, Jack and I had burned through his $10,000 royalty check in ten days and then scrounged for change to buy two Big Macs for a dollar on Big Mac Mondays. Every last dollar was feeding our drug use. I scammed Western Union to send myself money from my dad's credit card number I'd written down, and when he caught me, I said someone must have impersonated me. I pawned my computer, printer, television, DVD player, three guitars, two amps, my great-grandmother's wedding ring, and countless pieces of jewelry. I sold thousands of dollars' worth of clothing, shoes, records, books, furniture, my grandmother's clown collection, and, oh yeah, a Chagall painting.

Yet right then, sitting in my car on Valentine's Day, with the broken window, a soggy cigarette in my mouth and a wet arm,

I felt myself sinking my way to death in a new way. Wasn't that what this dance with addiction was—a long passive road to suicide? I felt like a fool for not just ending it all. *Why can't I just turn the key in the ignition, push the pedal all the way down, and plow through the cars and walls and trees and sidewalks of Los Angeles, until there is nothing left of me?*

Spitting the cigarette out the window, I slapped the side of my face, grabbed the "I see you" bracelet and the rest of the jewelry, and buzzed Pedro. Pedro was one of our crack dealers. The compulsion for crack led me to skipping the pawnshop altogether, arming myself with anything I thought he might accept as a trade. It didn't always work.

Pedro's apartment smelled like rice and beer, and he asked me to sit down. He loved the bracelet and put it on, wanted to keep it for himself, and I felt sick seeing it there on his arm next to his MS-13 tattoo. Before I left, he asked, "Are you okay? You gotta slow down a little, baby girl."

I felt even worse now. *What kind of drug dealer tells you to slow down?* And then I remembered that he was the second dealer to say that to me.

I left with a handful of rocks and returned to my car. It rained harder, and I couldn't stop myself from crying. The city wept with me. My cries became guttural, escaping the open window to a sleepy city that didn't respond. *You're a worthless piece of shit. You're a whore. You're a junkie. You're a monster. You lie. You steal. You fuck. You killed your baby. Nobody believes in you. Nobody loves you. Nobody sees you.*

I drove past a wall on the corner of Hollywood Boulevard and La Brea. I had hit that wall when I was sixteen in a minor car accident. *I could do it, end it, now. Push the fucking pedal.* The only thing that kept me driving straight, past the wall, past that ending, was the thought I might accidentally kill someone else in the process.

I returned home to find Jack passed out on the floor. I left him there and smoked a couple of rocks and went up to the roof of my building. I leaned against the low perimeter wall, looking down on Hollywood. Through the mist, against the lights of the city, I saw the corpse baby in a yellow shirt—floating, bloated, blue, carrying pieces of the sea—just out of reach. I wanted to reach her. I leaned my torso farther over the edge of the wall and felt it press against my stomach. *I could just lean forward, a little more.* I stuck my arms out and felt the outside of the wall. I shut my eyes, taking a deep breath that made my chest rattle.

"Hello…" A voice sounded behind me.

I was startled and spun around to see Bob, the building's security guard, shining a flashlight toward me.

"What are you doing up here?"

"Hey, Bob, I was just getting some air."

"Someone called and said you were close to the edge, leaning over the ledge there. I don't want you to slip."

I laughed. I wanted to tell him that the edge was the only place I existed anymore. "Oh, sorry. I didn't even see anyone else up here."

"Well, why don't you head back to your apartment. The roof is closed after eleven."

"Yeah. Yes, of course. Sorry."

We rode the elevator down in uncomfortable silence, my clothes soaked with mist and sweat. I watched Bob and his big round white face glance at me quickly and look away. I wondered who reported me and I imagined that it was the porn star with the mustache, who parked next to me and had been watching my quick descent, or maybe the dwarf actor, who lived down the hall. The absurdity of Los Angeles and the absurdity of it all made me laugh and I knew the security guard must have thought I was crazy. I went back to my apartment and smoked more crack.

At 6:00 a.m., I called Pete but hung up. At 7:00 a.m., I called Pete and hung up again. At 8:00 a.m., Pete called me back, and I didn't pick up. He left a message. At 9:00 a.m., I fell asleep. At

11:00 a.m., I woke up and my stomach was cramping, and I knew I was getting sick—again, already—and I didn't have enough dope to get well. Jack was up and making a pile of things to pawn. The pile was pretty pathetic. He left to go to his place, to see if he had a check or something better to pawn, and I called Pete. Pete was the only person I could think of to call. Diana was sober. No one else knew I was using. They suspected, but they didn't know. But more than that, Pete *knew me*—the light parts and the dark parts, too.

"Hello?"

"It's me," I said.

"Are you okay?"

"No."

We waited each other out in silence. Pete caved. "Well, what's going on?"

"I'm sick."

I heard him sigh softly.

"I'm strung out. I don't have even one dollar, and I have to get well. I've got class at four." The fact that I thought getting to class was ever going to happen was laughable. But I wasn't laughing. I started to cry.

He was silent, letting me cry. My tears were sincere, but I also knew they'd help get me what I needed. I wanted help, but I also didn't want help. I was so tired.

"Go to my apartment. There's a spare key under the pot next to the door for the housekeeper. Go into my room, the first door past the living room, and in the top dresser drawer, there should be some money there. There's not much, maybe $100."

I nodded, but he couldn't hear me. I took down the address.

"Don't ever ask me to do this again. I'm here for you. I'll be here for you. But I'm not gonna help you get high again."

"Pete…" I couldn't get anything else out. I silently choked on tears, on words, on feelings, on everything. "I won't. Thank you."

After we hung up, I showered and put on an old blue sweat-shirt that once belonged to Pete and jeans—my skinny jeans, which were now my baggy jeans. The rattle in my chest was worse and I felt shivery. The dope-sickness was settling in, spreading its way to every corner of my body.

By the time I found a parking spot near the apartment, I was clammy and shaky and dry heaving.

I'd never been inside this apartment. It wasn't actually Pete's apartment. He'd been staying there while his friend David was out of town. Pete didn't get a place right after we broke up. He went out of town for work and had been staying with friends and house-sitting, figuring out where he wanted to be. I found the building, which looked exactly like every other Spanish-style fourplex in the Miracle Mile. The key was where he said it would be.

Being inside David's apartment was strange. I didn't know him that well. It was a nice apartment, and it was dark with the shades drawn. It felt safe because no one was home. I headed into the guest room, opened the top drawer of the dresser, and found exactly $100 folded in the corner, next to Pete's boxers, five $20 bills. It smelled like Pete in there—the lavender Tancho stick he used in his hair and Gitanes cigarettes—and the smell shook me.

One of his shirts was on the edge of the bed—the blue plaid one. He might have been wearing it the first time we spoke, or the first night we split a Burst of Blue shake at Swingers, or the first night we sat in the rain in his car listening to "Cure for Pain" by Morphine and he kissed me. When I was with Pete, I believed we could escape LA together; I believed I could let him love me; I believed we could have a life together; and I believed it was possible for me.

I lay down on the bed shivering. Every muscle in my body seemed to be on the verge of contracting, like having restless leg syndrome all over. I held his shirt to my face and inhaled and smelled more of him, past the lavender Tancho and the

Gitanes, past the cloth, into the scent of him—the one that came out his pores, the one that slept next to me for two and a half years, the one I let go of. My stomach cramped in waves sharp and strong, and I curled myself into a ball. I didn't know which I wanted more of—his scent or heroin. The muted yellow light in the room soothed me, the smell of Pete in the air around me soothed me, the blue plaid cotton against my skin soothed me.

But the pull of heroin was stronger.

I put the blue plaid shirt back on the edge of the bed, put the key back underneath the pot, and I left to score from Gaela.

The next morning, Jack and I went to see Dr. D, an MD who specialized in medical detox. In other words, he prescribed drugs to help wean people off heroin. I'd seen him before, maybe five or six times. It was hard for me to tell if the drugs he prescribed helped.

The waiting room was filled with regular people, mostly older, mostly not there for Dr. D's bag of tricks—"alternative" opiates and muscle relaxers and antianxiety meds and sleeping pills and tranquilizers. *But shit*, I saw Ray, a musician friend I knew from twelve-step meetings. *I thought he was on tour.* We gave each other an uncomfortable nod hello and *oh, how funny, we're both here just for a regular old checkup.* We silently agreed to believe our parallel lies.

I sat on my hands in the waiting room on the third floor of that inconspicuous medical building and counted while I held my breath. I looked at the window on the far side of the room, wondering if I could run fast and open it and jump out without anyone stopping me. I studied the faces in the room. An old woman in a pale blue sweater stared at me. I'd been holding my breath for so long, when I exhaled the air came out with sound and force. Jack startled out of his half nod and glared at me.

I couldn't catch my breath. I walked up to the reception desk and asked for the key to the bathroom. As the receptionist handed it to me, she looked down at my hand and then away, which made me look, too. I'd been picking at the skin on my hand and had rows of tiny nail marks scrawled into me like some secret code.

Jack and I had decided that we'd start our kick that day, or more precisely, I decided, and he agreed. We waited to get our scripts filled in the lobby pharmacy that smelled like Band-Aids. A woman walked in with a sleeping baby, snug against her chest in a carrier. I shifted my weight on the hard orange plastic chair in the pharmacy and shut my eyes. But all I saw when I did was the dead baby, my dead baby. *She's wearing a yellow shirt and I can't remember her name.* I hadn't told Jack about my visions of the corpse baby or the time spent on the ledge or the invisible gun in my invisible pocket or the growing fear that I was going crazy. I knew something had to stop me, whether it was detoxing or the ledge or the box cutter or a wall. Something *had to* stop me—I knew I wouldn't or couldn't stop chasing that low until something with real force did.

We'd done our last bit of dope that morning. We headed straight home from Dr. D's to take as much as we could of his replacement drugs and hoped we'd make it through.

By 11:30 p.m., Jack was curled up in a ball on the floor. I lay on the couch and looked at him. *I detest him.* I detested him for having no visible reaction to the abortion. I detested him because he didn't have to see the corpse baby all day, every day. I detested him because he was weak. I detested him because he was with me. I detested him because he didn't really know me at all. He didn't see me. None of this was really his fault, so I detested me a little more.

Around midnight, Jack got up and called Gaela. He left, scored some dope, and we got well enough to sleep for a few hours. By 10:00 a.m. the next day, he was up and panicking, and I knew I couldn't keep doing this for one more second. I knew

I had two choices—go to the roof with my corpse baby and her yellow shirt and walk right to the edge and jump, or make a call.

Jack left to pawn his last guitar, and I called Pete. He answered.

"Pete, help. Please, help."

"Where are you?"

"I'm home. Can you come get me?"

He paused and said, "I'm not going to be able to come for a couple hours. Stay by the phone. I'll call you right back."

While I waited for Pete to call me back, I started to pack a bag, with an assortment of items that made no sense at all—a bikini, a dress, boots, jeans, a tank top, a pashmina, some makeup, and my school books for classes I never attended. I started to write a note to leave for Jack. My cell phone rang.

"Hey, okay, Diana is coming to get you, right now. I want you to go with her to her place, and I'm gonna pick you up in a few hours. Okay?"

"Okay. I'm sorry, Pete. I'm so fucking sorry."

"Just go with Diana when she comes. I'll see you soon."

Diana showed up twenty minutes later. When I opened the door, she started crying. She looked good, healthy, sober. I could see from her reaction how fucking terrible I looked. She went through my bag and grabbed some underwear for me, which I'd forgotten to pack.

"It's time to go," she said.

I finished writing my note for Jack just as he opened the front door. He saw Diana; he saw my bag.

"What are you doing?"

"I'm sorry. I can't do this anymore," I said or maybe whispered.

"What are you talking about? We'll kick together, we just need to get through the weekend. Come on, don't go. Baby, Zingo, I got dope."

He showed me the lump of tar in his hand. I saw Diana in my periphery, clutching her keys and my bag, breathing rapidly.

That familiar smell—shoe polish and vinegar and something sweetly rotten—grabbed hold of me and I gagged. I knew if I took a few hits, the dope-sickness that was running under my skin like an army of tiny knives would go away. The first couple of hits would be awful. I'd probably throw up, but then relief. I flashed through my options. Inhale. Jump. Leave.

"Erin, let's go," Diana said.

Jack was sick and wasted no time getting well. He plopped a piece of tar onto tinfoil, lit the bottom, and inhaled.

"Here," he said, shoving it into my hand as he exhaled.

The tinfoil fell to the ground. I shut my eyes. I heard the crinkle of the tinfoil being picked up, the click of the lighter, the sound of the tar bubbling up, and Jack inhaling—sickly sweet poisonous smoke. I was pulled in opposing directions.

"Erin, let's go. Now. Now, Erin."

Diana's quaking voice pulled harder. She grabbed my hand and we left, Jack yelling behind us. His voice sounded like it was underwater and I held my breath all the way to the elevator. When we got to Diana's car, I realized she was shaking, I realized she only had six months clean, I realized how fucked up that whole situation must have been for her.

She sat on the curb in front of her car and lit a cigarette. The hazy winter sunshine felt oppressive and I'd forgotten my sunglasses. I squinted and swayed, unsure of how I was standing. Diana looked up at me and then rummaged through her purse. "Here," she said, shoving a pair of sunglasses in my hand.

"Diana, I'm so sorry. I'm so, so sorry."

"I don't want you to die, Erin."

On the drive to her place, Diana was uncharacteristically silent and I chain-smoked. She'd moved to a new apartment, not far from where Pete had been staying. I asked to take a shower. As the water heated up, I looked at myself in the mirror, but this time I really looked, in a way I hadn't done in a very long time. I saw how badly I needed to pluck my eyebrows; I saw how I'd destroyed my skin by picking at it. I saw how drawn my face was, how sallow my skin was. I saw me. I saw every broken little piece. I saw how clearly strung out I looked. I saw it in my face—the months of guilt about having the abortion, feeling like a bad feminist for feeling remorse over it.

I'm pro-choice. I couldn't have that baby. But why couldn't I have her? Some part of me wanted that baby, not because I wanted a family with Jack, but because I wanted to love her. I wanted to protect her. *You could never be somebody's mother.* I saw it in my eyes—the belief I was too broken to be a mom. *They know you're a junkie, but they can't know you're crazy. They can't know you've been holding your breath, counting the seconds, leaving your body since you were four years old. They can't know. They won't believe you.* I felt worse still because I knew that I pushed away everyone who loved me—*because how could they love a monster?*

I got in the shower, and I let myself breathe. When I was done breathing and washing, I got out and plucked my eyebrows and put on some makeup and got dressed and sat in the kitchen with Diana, who made me some tea and toast. She held my hand. At dusk, there was a knock at the front door. I knew it was Pete. I couldn't hear what they were saying when Diana answered the door. I heard outlines of their voices and soft laughter. I wondered what was funny.

With the light behind him, Pete's tall, glowing frame stopped in the doorway to the kitchen. I took a deep breath and held it in, looking down. I looked so bad; I felt embarrassed. But he'd seen me through worse, hadn't he? I looked up again at his kind face, his cheekbones, his wheaten hair. I exhaled.

"Are you ready to go?"

I nodded. He walked over and took my hand, helping me up. I gave him an awkward hug, pressing my face into the side of his blue plaid shirt, once again taking in his scent.

Diana walked us to Pete's car and I got inside. They talked for what seemed like a long time and I couldn't hear what they were saying, but I heard the concern in their muffled tones.

Pete picked up Chinese food from Mandarette. I hadn't eaten there since we broke up. It was one of "our places." After, Pete drove us to his friend Lance's house, where he was house-sitting that weekend. Lance lived in a beautiful Spanish house in Benedict Canyon, with two huge adorable slobbering dogs. *I don't deserve to be here. I don't deserve Pete's kindness.* He tried to get me to eat a little, and I managed to choke down some plain white rice. I'd left my Dr. D pills with Jack and I was feeling sick. Pete put me to bed and I asked him to hold me and he did.

"Pete?"

"Yeah?"

"I've never hated myself more."

"It's gonna be okay, Erin."

"You don't know, Pete. You don't know."

I inched toward the wall, my forehead resting on the cool stucco.

"I had an abortion. And I know it was the right thing to do, but I fucking hate myself for it. That dead baby is with me all the time."

He held me, squeezing his arms around my body.

I went on to tell him about Juan's cousin and Providence and Whitey's twelve-year-old-nephew and my dad and the pawnshop and the ledge on the roof of my building.

He turned me around.

"How can you even look at me?"

"I will always love you. No matter what."

"I'm so scared."

Pete kissed my forehead, stroking my hair softly, and repeated, "It's gonna be okay."

Some microscopic piece of me believed him, and it was enough to get me through the night.

The next morning, after a rough night of cramping and throwing up and crying and shaking, I sat up and spoke words that came out of my mouth before my brain knew what was happening: "I want to go to rehab."

"I will do whatever you need me to do."

Pete called my insurance company and then called a rehab in Pasadena that I'd taken Nate to once before. I closed my eyes and imagined it waiting for me—serene and woodsy, a place to heal. He called Diana. And then he called my mom. After he spoke to her, I got on the phone. She was calm and we made a plan for her to come pick me up at Diana's and drive me to Pasadena.

Waiting for my mom later at Diana's, I lay on the floor, looking up at Pete and Diana sitting on the couch. Diana's living room had big beautiful wooden beams on the ceiling, and I looked at the beams and back at their faces. *These two people love me.* Diana's cat came and sat on me and purred. I was cold and clammy and my heart was racing, but I looked at Pete's eyes, the kindest eyes, and he was looking right at me. *I know he sees me.* That gave me the glimmer of hope I needed to get in the car with my mom.

CHAPTER 20
"You Can't Trust Water"
February 18, 2001

You can't trust water: Even a straight stick turns crooked in it.
—W. C. Fields

The lobby reminded me of a rustic lodge, maybe in Big Bear. Later, you can go skiing and come back and get in the hot tub and rest your bones and look at the stars, because you can see the stars here at night in the mountains. But we were not in the mountains. We were in Pasadena, and I was awaiting intake in the lobby of a behavioral health hospital.

The lighting was soft, and I smelled potpourri but also underneath it a slightly antiseptic smell. I had felt every variety of despair, fear, anger, sadness, and so much shame in the past three and a half months. Now, in that woodsy lobby, I felt a combination of tiredness, exhaustion, and flatness. And I was okay with it. I'd surrendered. Yes, my stomach was slam-dancing, and my body was a knot of seized muscle, and I was sweaty and light-headed, and everything was too loud and too smelly and too much. At the center of it all I was relieved. That relief carried magic, a magic that made the withdrawal symptoms bearable.

"Erin, come in," the counselor called from the edge of the hallway.

My mom smiled at me, watery eyed, and squeezed my hand. I was glad she was there. I knew that she loved me—in a way I hadn't felt in years.

The counselor, an aging hippie with long ash-blond hair who hummed while she walked, led us into her office and I was immediately distracted by the greeting cards plastered all over the wall behind her desk. I wondered what the point was of having them behind her where she couldn't see them.

The counselor told us her name, twice, but I couldn't remember it, and this missing information was distracting as she asked me a series of questions. I answered without emotion, plainly, honestly—detailing my drug history, bringing her up to the present day.

"When was the last time you used?"

"Friday night. Wait, no, I guess the middle of the night or early morning Saturday."

"In the past week, what drugs have you taken?"

"Heroin, crack, Norco, Xanax, Flexeril."

Lynne? Is her name Lynne? Lonnie?

"Were you using intravenously?"

"No, I mean not for a couple years. I've been smoking mostly."

She looks more like a Lynne than a Lonnie. Maybe her name doesn't even start with L.

"In the past thirty days, how often did you use each of these substances?"

"How often? I mean, all the time. Constantly. Or not the pills, that was really just the last week or few days. But with heroin and crack—pretty much twenty-four hours a day."

I noticed Mom tighten her face and shoulders and shift in her seat. My ears began to ring, and the room that had felt cozy became stifling and the person answering the counselor's questions disconnected from me. I hardly knew her.

After the interview, we waited in the lobby for someone from "down the hill" to come get me. Down the hill was where the drug addicts were, except for those with severe dual diagnoses, who needed to stay here in the main building, the hospital part.

I wondered about Jack. I wondered if he knew where I was, if he was still getting high, if he'd dared to call Diana or, worse, Pete. I was so grateful to both of them. What if Pete hadn't answered the phone? What if Diana had said no, she couldn't come get me? Where would I be without their support? *Pete.* I felt waves of old regret. I missed him. I had missed him every day since we broke up. My sadness settled over me, at odds with the relief I'd felt earlier.

A woman appeared before us—Marcy, a younger version of the counselor maybe named Lynne. I panicked a little when I hugged my mom goodbye, but I went with Marcy. I picked up my small black duffel bag—the bag I'd put a bikini in and thankfully Diana replaced with underwear—and I followed Marcy.

Down the hill was comprised of cottages. There was the main cottage, where the detox beds were, and the nurses' station and a living room. Outside, there was a patio with chairs and a payphone, and a group of men and women were smoking. They smiled and nodded at me as I walked inside, and one guy looked familiar. The other cottages a little farther off were where the "residents" lived during their stay. They looked like little log cabins, connected in clustered groups of four, surrounded by pine trees and green grass. I noticed everything was a little damp from the rain.

The last time I had been to this facility, I was visiting Nate and thought, *It's so peaceful and woodsy, like camp.* Getting my temporary bed in the detox ward with a plastic mattress, within view of the nurses' station, it felt a little less like camp and a little more like a sanitarium.

I got checked in and answered more of the same questions. The male nurse with pitted tawny skin and slicked-back hair gave me a small paper cup of water and an even smaller cup with some detox meds.

"You can go out on the patio for a little before bedtime," he said.

"Thanks," I said as I tried to get the pills down.

Outside, I met the others. Much like at my first rehab, they were mostly men, only two other women. The guy who looked familiar turned out to be a singer-songwriter I adored with a lot of mostly underground acclaim. It wasn't exactly surprising to see him there because his drug use was pretty well documented. There was the country singer who I'd never heard of, but it seemed like other people had. There was the blonde hummingbird—she moved so fast constantly, I was fairly sure she was on something like meth. There was the all-American football player who had a promising college career. He loved football, but he loved Oxy and cocaine a little more. There was the famous funk singer whose songs I knew from my parents' disco parties. He was clearly the patriarch but was leaving the next day and everyone was bummed about it.

"You see that bungalow there," the funk singer said with a twinkle in his eyes, pointing to the one closest to us, the one with the extra wide door. "That was made for W. C. Fields when he came here to dry out. And we've all heard him."

"Heard him?" I asked, taking a long drag of my Parliament cigarette.

"Oh yeah, his ghost."

"He died here," said the hummingbird.

I was struck by what an LA moment this was.

"It's not his ghost. It's the damn old pipes," said Sandy.

Everyone laughed. I immediately liked Sandy. She was forty, though she looked twenty, with long golden corkscrew curls and bright eyes. She instantly felt like an anchor, made me feel like I was going to be okay there.

There were two more campers in detox beds, but no one had seen them yet. And then there were more up the hill in the mental hospital—the dual diagnoses campers. I started to feel weak and must have looked it, too.

"Hey, you need to sit down," said Sandy, patting the chair next to her.

"So, what are you in for?" asked the funk singer.

Before I had a chance to answer, the hummingbird started. "I don't really have a problem. I just did a little crystal, you know, occasionally."

I swore I could see her tiny wings flapping.

"Heroin, mostly," I said.

"Pills," said the football player.

"Yup, pills. Oxy," said the country singer.

"Heroin, but mostly life," said the singer-songwriter.

"Everything," said the funk singer, and everyone laughed.

Sandy went last. "Heroin, too. And this is the first time I've been clean for more than five consecutive days in fifteen years."

The weight of what she said got the ringing in my ears going again.

"What day are you on?" asked the funk singer.

"Day two, I guess."

"You look pretty good for being on day two, girl."

"Thanks, but I think you might need new glasses."

Everyone laughed again. I laughed, too, which was a surprise. The February air was cool and moist, and despite the slightly institutional aura coming off the main cottage, I could almost pretend I was at camp.

"All right, ladies and gents, it's time to head back to your cottages," came a voice from behind us.

Marcy's announcement broke the illusion. This was not camp. My detox room was neither woodsy nor peaceful. The plastic mattress amplified how sweaty I was, and I could hear the other two detoxers, who I'd yet to see, coughing, getting up to use the bathroom, pleading with the nurse. I smelled that horrid rotten scent coming out of me along with Lysol and dampness in my small room, and I started to panic a little.

"Can I please go outside for a minute? I think I'm having a panic attack," I said to the male nurse.

"Yeah, go on then but don't leave the patio."

I sat down on one of the cold metal chairs and took a deep breath, my chest rattling.

"I think we're going to need to get you an inhaler. Sounds like asthma."

Marcy appeared and sat down beside me.

"Oh, I don't think I have asthma," I said.

"Well, you've been smoking a lot, right?"

"Yeah, I guess."

I had been smoking a lot, constantly—inhaling nicotine, crack, heroin—and my chest had felt congested for weeks. Marcy was a nail-biter, and I watched her look at her nails, contemplate, and bite a little cuticle, and then sit on her hands. She talked a little about the weather and knitting and her niece. She went inside and came back with a grape soda. She poured some into a Dixie cup and handed it to me. The smell of grape soda covered all the other smells. I could see the country singer and the football player on the porch of the W. C. Fields cottage, the one with the wide door. I wondered if that story was true. The country singer was playing guitar. I heard a woman laugh. Maybe it was Sandy laughing. Maybe this *was* camp.

After two days in the detox room, I moved into a cottage with Sandy as my roommate. Our cottage shared walls with the W. C. Fields cottage, and his ghost, or those awful old pipes, made noise every night. It rained while I was there, almost every day, and Sandy and I played cards and smoked on the porch and talked about the brooding new guy we nicknamed Dracula, who played the piano all the time in the main cottage and barely spoke to any of us. We watched *Harold and Maude* over and over. It was the one DVD Sandy brought with her, and every time Cat Stevens started singing, "Trouble..." I'd clench my jaw in a pointless attempt to stop the tears.

Our meals were served up in the cafeteria in the main building with the hospital. I hated being up there. The patients *up there* scared me. I was scared of their mental illness. I was scared of what it would be like in a locked unit, of shuffling in a bathrobe to the cafeteria, of being overmedicated or given ECT and losing memory, of being labeled crazy. I was afraid of being near the ward because I knew it wouldn't take much for me to be right there with them. I knew I was just as broken. Ever since I was small, I'd had this great fear that one day I'd be locked away. One day, everyone would figure out how different I was, how crazy I was, and they'd lock me up and I'd die there. Getting help and going to rehab had always been overshadowed by the fear of being committed.

Jack and CeCe came to visit. The day I'd checked into rehab, Jack had gone to stay with her and kick on her couch. We sat on the patio. CeCe did most of the talking, and Jack sat with his hands in his leather jacket and looked down a lot. When CeCe went to use the bathroom, he looked up.

"God, Zingo, I'm so sorry, about everything," he said, his blue eyes wide and shining and contrite.

"No, it's not... You don't have to apologize to me. I did this. You didn't do this to me." I leaned forward and hugged him, and he put his face in my neck, and I could feel his tears.

He pulled back and said, "I think I need to go back to Chicago for a while. Stay with my parents. Just get my head together."

"I think that's a good idea," I said, nodding.

I had other visitors, too. Sunny came to see me. She brought her six-month-old, whom I hadn't met yet, and vegetarian sandwiches from Say Cheese in Silverlake. Her baby was asleep. We lay her down on my bed and sat on Sandy's bed and had a picnic.

Mary came to see me, too. Mary was a woman I'd known since early sobriety. She was a few years older than me, had a young daughter, and was going through a divorce. We were both tall and thin and had both chopped off our dark hair into pixie cuts. People used to always confuse us for each other, said we looked so much alike. This was a compliment. Mary was beautiful, and I didn't see the same beauty in me. Pete had run into her at a twelve-step meeting and told her where I was and asked her if she could visit me, said I needed some female support. She showed up on a dark Sunday in the pouring rain. When I saw her, I burst into tears—a flood of emotions that took me by surprise. I asked her if she would be my sponsor. She said yes.

This second trip to rehab was very different than my first one three and a half years earlier. I didn't have the same fears; I knew sobriety was possible. But I had new fears. I worried I'd do this over and over, that I would relapse again and again. I was scared of the ledge of the roof and the box cutter and the myriad other ways I'd fantasized about killing myself. I was petrified that I would never be able to fully address what was wrong with me, what made me want to get low in the first place.

After the funk singer left, the singer-songwriter did, too. The country singer and the football player left, and they came back to an outpatient group high, and it broke my heart. We never saw the football player again, but the country singer came back and started over in detox again, determined to get it right, determined to go back to Nashville and be a husband and father and salvage his career. Within three years, both the funk singer and singer-songwriter would be dead. And there would be so many more drug-related deaths. Addiction spares no one. Making it out is akin to winning the lottery, even when you have the resources and access for help. I knew this; I wanted to make it out, but my faith that I could wavered from day to day.

What was majorly different this time—what hadn't fully been discussed during my first trip to rehab—was my mental health. One of the doctors who ran the program was Dr. Drew, the doctor I'd listened to on *Loveline* all those years before. He and another doctor, Dr. P, oversaw the program. Dr. Drew ran some of the family group meetings, and he was better at explaining addiction to family members than anyone I'd ever heard. He talked about the science of addiction as a brain disorder. He emphasized that addiction was not the result of a moral failing. He explained how childhood trauma was rocket fuel for addiction. He talked about the commonality of the trifecta—childhood trauma, substance use, and a psychiatric disorder. Listening to Dr. Drew made me feel less scared about facing mental illness.

Meanwhile, Dr. P guided me in addressing those mental health issues. We talked about the sexual abuse. We talked about my long-standing struggle with wanting to kill myself. We talked about borderline personality disorder and rapid cycling bipolar disorder, which he said couldn't really be determined until my body and brain had time to come back to stasis without narcotics. He got me back on the antidepressant Wellbutrin and back in therapy under the care of a psychiatrist.

My parents came to family groups—my mom and dad and my stepdad, too. They were there for me, once more. It was decided that we'd sell my condo, and I never stepped foot in it again. My parents moved my things into storage, and when I transitioned from inpatient to outpatient, I moved in with my mom and stepdad. My first weekend at Mom's, Dad flew in to see me.

We went through my pawn tickets, the ones that hadn't already been lost, and he and I went to both pawnshops and retrieved what we could. I returned the stolen jewelry we could save to my mother, things she hadn't even known were missing. My grandmother's jade pendant, however, was lost. I'd defaulted on the ticket, and it had already sold. She was devastated. She tried to get the information on who bought it. She continued to call pawnshops to see if maybe it would turn up somewhere else. She wasn't mad at me—that wasn't how she expressed what she felt—but she was crushed that it was gone. I felt horribly about it; I still do. That jade pendant is emblematic of the wreckage we leave behind in the wake of addiction. That wreckage can be so hard to face, to shake out the shame it carries, but the only way out is through it.

One night, after being at my mom's for a couple of weeks, I found my stepdad's acoustic guitar in a closet. On nights when I couldn't sleep, I started playing, trying to remember the basic chords Jack had taught me the year before. And I started writing songs even though I didn't know what I was doing. The music did something for me. I started keeping a journal again and wrote song lyrics. This renewed connection to writing and expression was a gift. It was that elusive feeling one gets from creating something, from reflecting on the human experience, that brings a type of satisfaction like nothing else can. I believed in living again. I believed that maybe I could stay off drugs. I believed that maybe I could be happy.

CHAPTER 21
Flightless
September 8, 2001

"Oh God, Pete's here. And he's with her," I whispered into Mary's ear, clutching her arm. We were at an after-party for a friend's gallery opening in a loft in downtown LA. I knew Pete would be there, but seeing him walk in with Ava still felt like a sucker punch.

Out of the corner of my eye, I saw Michael looking at me. Michael was this odd guy who had been pursuing me that summer. I wasn't exactly attracted to him, but he was interesting. He was older than me—I wasn't sure by how much. He looked like the grunge version of Daniel Day-Lewis, and he seemed to know everyone, or everyone seemed to know him. I'd heard about him for years—he had some large, macabre house that everyone had lived in at one time or another, he was a record producer, and he was a total womanizer.

Mary and I ducked around the corner. I needed to prepare myself before I said hello to Pete.

In the weeks and months after treatment, I'd spent my days playing guitar, going to many, many twelve-step meetings, thrift store shopping, spending most of my time with Mary. She had quickly morphed from sponsor to best friend. Since getting sober, I'd tried once again to reconcile with Pete. In April, I wrote him a very long letter, apologizing for the ways I'd let him down, asking him to consider trying again with me, telling him how much I loved him. I gave him the letter and asked him to meet me at Torung, a Thai restaurant on Hollywood Boulevard that we'd been to many times before.

I nervously shifted in the red vinyl booth as we made small talk about music and work and how our mothers were doing. I sucked down my Thai iced tea. The sugar made me antsy and sick to my stomach. I needed to know where his head was at.

"So, did you read my letter?" I asked, my voice cracking.

"Yeah, of course, I read it," he said, looking down and back up again. "Erin, you know I will always love you."

"I know," I said, cutting him off.

"But I can't go there again with you. It wouldn't be good. For either of us."

I clenched my jaw and pleaded with my eyes to cooperate. They were welling up. *Please don't cry, Erin. Please don't cry.*

"I have to go to the bathroom," I said, jerking up.

"Erin," Pete said and grabbed my hand.

"No, I'm okay. I'm not... I mean, I totally understand. I think I just needed to get it all out. You're right. Of course, you're right. I just really do have to go to the bathroom."

I locked the bathroom door behind me and let myself sob into the flimsy wood door.

The next week at a twelve-step meeting, Pete was there with a tall, very thin young woman. I'd come to find out this was Ava. She was newly sober, and they were dating. It took every ounce of actress energy in me to pretend that it didn't crush me to see them together.

Meanwhile, I was writing songs and playing music with Mary. We started a band and called ourselves the Gene Hackman Band because, well, we both loved Gene Hackman. I'd also started writing and playing music with another friend I'd met in meetings, Lyle. Lyle was tall and lanky and reminded me of a folksy version of Noel Gallagher from Oasis. Much as Jack had done the year before, Lyle encouraged me to write music. It didn't matter that I could barely play guitar, he said, I could write a song. We recorded a few songs and started to plan some live shows.

I felt resurrected by music, a creative outlet that gave me somewhere to put all the anxiety and insomnia and heartbreak.

Jack was still in Chicago but we talked frequently, and he invited me to come to Chicago, as a friend, and play a show with him, a memorial show for another musician who had died. Unfortunately, the trip did not go as planned. It became clear to me pretty quickly that Jack was using again. He was spending lots of time with a couple of other well-known Chicago-based musicians who were notorious for their heroin use. He vehemently denied it, until I found his stash, like I had the year before, carelessly left inside a compact mirror in the bathroom. By my fourth day there, we were barely speaking. Under my repulsion for Jack and his drug use, I felt the old familiar pull toward an exit that heroin could provide.

Jack dragged me in the stifling afternoon heat of the city to meet up with the singer of a band and a record label guy. We met them in an old dark bar that was classic Chicago. My cell phone rang and I excused myself to take the call. While outside on the phone, I was mugged. I fought the guy. He got my purse but I got his wallet, along with his ID, social security card, and a folded-up copy of his birth certificate. In exchange, he got from my bag $5 and credit cards that I immediately shut off. Still, the mugging shook me and made me feel unsafe. It was hot, I was miserable, and I wanted to get high.

"I want to get high," I said to Jack.

"What?"

"I want to get high."

"Are you sure?"

"I'm sure."

This was a relapse I didn't see coming or give much thought about. Looking back, I should have left Chicago when I found out Jack was using. But I didn't. Relapses like this one are the hardest to understand. But they show just how powerful addiction can be. The impulse can take the wheel and temporarily erase the memory of just how bad things were only a few months prior. Without time and practice and tools, relapse is a very high probability for people in recovery. It's why aftercare is crucial. It's why support groups and mental health care are essential. I never should have gone to Chicago in the first place and I certainly shouldn't have stayed.

For the next three days, we snorted heroin and had sex and roamed the city. It felt fun and sexy and like a relief—for the first two days. On the last day, we fought and argued and he threw a phone at me. I got on a plane later that day and flew home. I didn't tell anyone what happened. Like I'd done so many times before, I relapsed and then pretended it didn't happen. When I got home, I resumed going to meetings and playing music and hanging out with my sober friends.

By September, I was staying sober. I was also feeling hyper and cagey, like I might go off the rails. More specifically, I felt boy crazy. As it had in the past, sex or love or both became an alluring and easy way to fill the hole that heroin left. Michael—the weird record producer who wore hats all the time—kept asking me out. I'd started hanging out with a couple of other guys—both musicians—in that blurry territory, the one where you can pretend you might not know if you're dating or just friends. I'd given up on Jack, who was thankfully in rehab again in LA. But I was still heartbroken over Pete and trying to pretend that I wasn't.

Michael walked up to Mary and me. "What are you two troublemakers whispering about?"

"Do you really want to know?" I asked.

"Yes."

"Well, my ex is here with his new girlfriend and I wasn't feeling real prepared to face them."

"Where are they?"

I pointed to the hallway and the three of us peered our heads gingerly around the wall. There they were.

"Come on," Michael said, and he took me by the hand, then whispered in my ear, "Pretend I said something hilarious."

I started laughing and we walked right past them and I pretended I didn't notice. We walked out onto the fire escape.

"Thank you," I said.

"He was totally checking you out, wondering who the mysterious man was holding your hand."

"Ha!"

Michael and I stood there for a long time, talking about the weird dreams we'd been having, how it felt like earthquake weather, what music we'd been listening to, and where we would travel if we could go anywhere in the world.

On my way back inside, Mary grabbed my arm and said, "Erin, don't go there with Michael. It is *not* a good idea."

"I'm not going there," I said.

I came face-to-face with Pete on my way to the bathroom. Ava was across the room, talking to someone. We spoke for a few minutes. It was awkward and I could see Ava turn to look at us, repeatedly. *I have to let you go. I know.*

"What?" Pete said.

But I hadn't said anything. Maybe he felt it.

"Nothing, I just have to pee. It was good to see you. Take care."

I hugged him, and he kissed me on the neck, and a shiver of sadness spread down my spine, and I went into the bathroom.

I was restless. I'd been tossing and turning after yet another night in a string of nights of strange and apocalyptic dreams that woke me up. Maybe it was the earthquake weather; maybe it was letting go of Pete.

"Erin. Erin, wake up. Wake up."

My roommate Alex was standing above me. His shaggy blond hair was messy from sleep, but he was wide-awake.

"What's up?" I asked.

"You need to come downstairs. Something happened in New York."

"Huh?"

"Just come downstairs."

It was barely 6:00 a.m., and we sat, mouths agape, watching the news. The North Tower of the World Trade Center had been hit. As we sat, trying to figure out what we were looking at, a second plane hit the South Tower. Much like the rest of America, we were bewildered and scared and felt like the world was ending.

As the details were broadcast, I realized that the second plane was United Flight 175 from Boston to LA. *Fuck, is that my dad's plane? Is that the flight he was taking?* My dad was en route to LA the night before from Providence. The plane coming in was late, and he would miss his connection through Chicago. He'd left me a voice mail that he was coming out the next morning instead, on the first flight out of Boston. The floor dropped away from my feet as I scurried to get my cell phone.

I called Stacy, who was now my dad's wife. They'd married the weekend before. Now I had a stepmom and stepsister, and a new half sister, Anya. She didn't pick up. I left her a voice mail. I called my dad's cell next and left a message. I kept calling and leaving messages. I finally called Ken and Olga's house, where my dad usually stayed when he came to LA. Ken was his best friend. Olga answered the phone.

"Olga, is Ken there? I need to know what time my dad was getting in today."

"He's already here, troll. He got here late last night."

I immediately broke down, crying fat tears of relief. Fortunately for our family, as my dad was walking away from the gate
in Providence the night before, a gate agent called out after him.
The flight was landing. He would make the connection. He
wouldn't have to fly out of Boston the next morning. By pure
happenstance, he wasn't destined to be on Flight 175.

That evening, Alex and I went to a twelve-step meeting.
Afterward, we went to a diner with a bunch of other friends.
Everyone was in a state of shock, of paralysis, trying to figure
out what this all meant, what was going to happen next. As we
were leaving the diner, Michael was walking up the sidewalk.

"Hey," he said.

"Hi."

We stood in silence for a moment.

"What a mindfuck of a day, huh?" he said.

"I don't even know… I can't even process it."

"What are you doing?"

"Right now?"

"Yeah."

"Going home, I guess. I don't know."

"I have a better idea. Let's go for a walk. I know the perfect
place," he said.

I went with him. We drove into Hollywood and parked near
my old condo.

We walked up to the top of Runyon Canyon on the hiking
trail, mostly in silence. When we got to the top, we sat on a
bench and looked down at the quiet city below us, twinkling,
silent. There wasn't a plane in sight, but the sky held electricity,
a current that had been pulsing in the air around me for days.

We talked about music and whether or not the world was
ending. He turned to me. "So, do you like me yet?"

I laughed and said, "Like you? I mean, I don't really know you.
Sure, I like you. I'm not sure if I'm attracted to you, though."

He laughed back and said, "That's the thing about me—the thing women like. They're attracted and repulsed by me at the same time, and there's no stronger magnet than that."

He leaned over and kissed me. It was strange and sad and exhilarating and somehow magical.

We started sleeping together shortly after our first date on 9/11. I told him not to tell anyone we were together. Everyone had warned me not to get involved with him—Mary, my roommate Alex, and most of my friends. The fact that everyone told me to stay away from him is part of what pushed me toward him. Like a defiant child, I was sure I'd be the one *not* to get caught up in the messiness of feelings and Michael's womanizing. I was right—for a little while.

Michael was good at making people feel special and I was no exception. He cooked for me. He surprised me with guitar pedals and encouraged my songwriting. He invited me on 3:00 a.m. bike rides through the quiet mid-city streets of Los Angeles. He told me I had a sparkling soul. But I'd come to learn that his attention, how he made one person feel so special, could only last so long.

When Michael started pulling back, giving evasive answers to seemingly simple questions, I felt myself holding on tighter to something—to someone—that I didn't even think I wanted. I became jealous and suspicious and while he always denied that he was seeing anyone else, my gut knew otherwise. He was adept at making me feel like it was all in my head. The more he backed away, the more I held fast.

In November, I started a new job working for a nonprofit as a case manager for homeless youth. I got the job through Carmen, an acquaintance I knew from twelve-step meetings. She was small and fiery, with long dark hair and perfect eyebrows. The first time I'd met her was years before when she got up and spoke at a meeting about overdosing. I'd always remembered her because she was wearing green ski overalls and had just come from the hospital. Now she had a few years clean. We'd started hanging out after meetings. She was a few years younger than me, and we just clicked.

Shortly after I started the new job, Pete called me. He and Ava had relapsed and were using heroin together. He was strung out and reaching out for help, just as I had to him earlier that year.

"I need someplace to kick. I can't go to my mom's. Do you think... I mean..."

Before he could finish his question, I answered, "Of course you can come here. Where are you?"

I picked him up on a cold Friday night from a motel on Beverly Boulevard, not far from The Grove. He got in my car like a ghost—thin and sunken. I chatted on the ride back to my house, filling the silence, hoping that would put him at ease.

"I just started a new job. You remember that girl, Carmen? Well, I started working with her, doing outreach with homeless kids in Santa Monica."

"That's great, Erin. I think you'll be really good at it."

"Thanks. Yeah, I like it so far. The only thing that sucks is driving to Santa Monica."

He turned the music up. It was the Stones, "Torn and Frayed"—one of his favorites, and the song I had so often played because it reminded me of him. He turned it back down after a minute.

"I feel bad about leaving Ava there," he said.

"Did she know you were leaving?"

"Yeah. She didn't want me to go. But I just knew I couldn't get clean if we were together, you know?"

"I know."

We got home, and Pete took a shower and got into my bed. I went back out for some detox-friendly food: soup and Gatorade and bread for toast. He was in bad shape when I got back—sweaty and tossing and turning, his muscles contracting and releasing in spasms of withdrawal. He wouldn't eat.

"At least drink a little Gatorade," I said, sitting on the bed.

He pulled his weak body upright and leaned forward as I held the bottle for him to take a sip. "Thanks. Fuck. What did I do?" He looked at me, his eyes watery.

"It happens to the best of us," I said.

"I'm sweating so much," he said, pulling the damp T-shirt over his head and throwing it on the floor.

He took my hand and held it tightly, then pulled me toward him. I leaned into his chest and hugged him. His head dropped to rest heavy on my shoulder, and I smoothed his hair behind his ears.

While he was in the shower, I called Michael. He'd been acting aloof. I didn't know if I wanted to cling or run. Our phone call was short; he gave some vague explanation of where he was and what his plans were for the rest of the week. I hung up, agitated, and went out on the small balcony off my bedroom to smoke. I looked down at the twinkling lights in the distance, the gentle hum of the 5 Freeway in the distance. I tried to sort out what it was I felt for Michael and, what I thought was more important at the time, what he felt for me. *Am I falling for him?*

Pete and I slept curled into each other, in our underwear, forehead to forehead. He woke up frequently. We talked. Sometimes we kissed. I knew it wasn't a path back to each other. I knew the affection sprang from comfort more than love. But I'd be lying if I said I didn't still love him.

Ava had been calling Pete incessantly. The next morning, he asked if he could give her my number, if I could talk to her instead, to give her updates on how he was doing. That afternoon, she called me.

"Erin?" she said, garbled, through tears. "This is—"

"Hi, Ava."

"How is he?"

"He's okay. He's been trying to sleep, and we're going to a meeting later."

I didn't tell her that we'd held each other all night and kissed and that I wanted her to go away and leave him alone.

"Can I come to your house? Can I come see him?"

"I don't think that's a good idea. You need to take care of yourself and try to get healthy, and he needs to do the same thing. And I don't think, he doesn't think, you can do that if you're together."

She broke into large sobs. I'd despised her when they started dating, but I knew she was dope-sick, I knew that place, and my empathy overrode my jealousy.

"Ava, you're going to be okay. Pete's going to be okay."

"I don't want to lose him."

"You're not going to lose him, but you have to focus on getting some help yourself, okay?" I knew that was a lie. She was going to lose him.

"Please, please, I just need to see him. Can I come over after the meeting?"

"I will have him call you after the meeting, okay? And you need to get to one, too."

I took Pete to a meeting, and when we got out, he had several missed calls from Ava. He called her back on the way home. She was hysterical, and he told her she could come to see him.

We sat in the living room watching *The Sopranos* while we waited. It had started to rain. His phone rang. It was Ava. When he hung up the phone, he said, "She's here."

"Here?"

"At the top of the driveway. She doesn't want to come in. She wants me to come sit in her car."

"Okay."

"But I need to tell you something."

"What?"

"I'm pretty sure she brought dope. I don't think I should be alone with her."

"Okay, well, what are you asking me to do?"

"Can you go with me?"

"To her car?"

"Yeah."

Pete and I walked up the long steep drive to the top of the street, huddled under an umbrella. Her face fell when she saw me. I felt bad. She was as lost as I had been, maybe still was.

I stood back and let Pete talk to her through the window. I couldn't hear what they were saying. But I could hear her crying. Pete turned and started walking back to the house without me. Ava screamed for him to come back. I walked over to the car and knelt into the window, trying to stay dry under my crappy umbrella.

"Why won't he talk to me?" she said, sobbing into her hands, with her head on the steering wheel.

"He will. You just need to give him a little space right now. He feels like shit."

Her body shook as she cried. She looked tiny like a little field mouse. "I don't have anyone else. He's all I have. You don't understand," she said.

"I do understand, Ava. I do. I'm so sorry. I know how hard this is. Just give him space for a few days, okay? You can call me if you need to, but just let him have some space."

When I got back to the house, Pete was sitting on the porch, smoking.

"Thanks. I just couldn't. I don't know. I saw tinfoil in her lap, and I couldn't get in the car."

"No, you did the right thing."

In bed that night, Pete told me that he'd stolen from his mom, quite a bit—cash and gold and jewelry. She didn't know they were gone.

"How am I gonna tell her?"

"Don't worry about that right now."

I held Pete while he cried tears of shame and exhaustion and fear, the kind of tears I knew very well, the kind I'd shed when he'd held me so many times in the past.

"Do you want me to talk to her?"

"You would do that?"

"Yes. For you, yes."

Pete's mom and I had had a good relationship. I was closer to her than with any other boyfriend's mom, and we'd even stayed in touch after Pete and I broke up. I called her the next day and told her he was safe; he'd been clean for two days, he was going to meetings. She was so relieved. She hadn't been able to find him and had been terrified. Then I told her what he'd told me, that he'd stolen from her. She was understandably dismayed. She said that she loved him, she was relieved he was safe, but that he couldn't come back to live with her and she didn't want to talk with him yet.

I hung up the phone and went to find Pete, who was having a smoke on the porch. I sat down next to him and lit a cigarette.

"Did you talk to her?" he asked.

"Yeah. She loves you. She's glad you're okay."

He nodded his head, his eyes focused somewhere distant.

"You can stay here. As long as you need to," I said.

"I don't know. I mean, I don't think we should fall back into each other, do you?"

"Well, you don't have to live with me like my boyfriend. I am dating someone else, you know."

"I know."

"You can have the basement, as long as you need it."

I had a finished basement, with its own entrance, and it would become Pete's home for the foreseeable future.

"Thank you. You saved my life," he said.

I hugged him and squeezed his broad shoulders and whispered in his ear, "You saved mine, too."

While Michael was out of town, visiting his family in Las Vegas, I spent Christmas at my mom's. I wasn't alone. I brought Carmen, my roommate Alex, and Jack and Pete. Amazingly, we had a good time. A year before that, I'd been in relapse hell with Jack, pining for Pete. And there we were—friends—spending a holiday together.

After dinner, after we'd helped clean up, my friends and I sat in my mom's den, drinking coffee and telling stories. Jack told everyone about my airplane freak-out the year before when I thought I was going to get arrested. His imitation of me was spot-on. I laughed so hard that my ribs hurt. That laughter was healing, necessary. I sat on the arm of the brown leather arm-chair, next to Pete.

He put his hand on my leg and said, "I really needed that story." We looked at each other and burst into another fit of laughter.

"Mark Twain had it right," said Jack. "Tragedy plus time, man. That's what's funny."

CHAPTER 22
A Simple Line
2002

Michael returned from his trip in time for New Year's Eve. He was back to his original charming self, making me feel special and sparkly and I wanted more of that. Within a couple of weeks, he was once again alternating between being attentive and then disappearing. The back-and-forth was quickly making me lose my mind. I stopped taking Wellbutrin after he'd made a condescending comment about psych meds. He'd vanish, not call when he'd say he was going to, and then show up again, showering me with affection. I knew it was a game. I knew this was what everyone had warned me about, but I couldn't stop it. I couldn't stop myself from wanting him to want me.

Shortly after Valentine's Day, he ended things with me. I found out he'd been seeing someone else the entire time we'd been dating. Not just one someone, but many, and one of them was now his girlfriend. I felt crushed. *This is my karma*, I thought, *for all my shitty behavior in relationships.*

A deep depression began tightening around my neck. I felt paralyzed by it, suffocated. I started cutting myself again, digging my nails into my arms. I forced myself to stay still for minutes at a time, resisting the urge to jump out the window or grab a knife or ram my car into a wall. I hadn't used for months, not since Chicago with Jack. But heroin soon became all I could think about. I picked up the phone and called Diana.

"I'm gonna get high."

"What are you talking about?" she asked.

"I am going to get high today. If I don't, I'm gonna fucking kill myself."

We sat in silence for a minute on the phone.

"I'm coming over," she said.

We called Vanessa, Juan's ex-girlfriend, one of our old connections. An hour later, Diana and I were driving around with heroin and a box of Reynolds foil we bought at a 7-Eleven, trying to figure out where we should get high. We couldn't go to her place—her husband was there. We couldn't go to my place since my roommate Alex was home.

"I want to drive by my old house," I said.

"Okay."

Diana drove us through Glendale toward the foothills of the San Gabriel Mountains, back into the Verdugo Woodlands, up the broad street lined with oak trees that led to the small canyon where my childhood home sat. We parked in front, and I looked up at the towering white Spanish house, the twenty-eight red steps that led to the front door, the giant oak tree in the front yard, and the balcony off of my childhood bedroom.

I don't know why I needed to see it. Maybe because of the depression I was in, I needed to see where it had all started. Maybe I was looking for something I'd lost a long time ago. Maybe I thought I could go back to some before time, before it all went wrong.

"Let's go to Verdugo Park," I said, and Diana followed my directions to the park I used to play in as a kid.

We found a spot in a remote corner of a back parking lot, tore off some tinfoil, and relapsed together. I rolled down the window and let the heroin take hold of my body. I waited for the relief that it would bring, should bring, and it didn't happen. To cross that line again and to not have it work at all was crushing. And worse, once again, I'd dragged Diana down with me.

When I got home later, Carmen and Pete were watching a movie. They'd gone to a twelve-step meeting I was supposed to be at. I said I was tired and needed a shower. I went upstairs and smoked more heroin. The relief still didn't come. But I was high, and now I needed to hide it.

I sat on the couch next to Pete, and I could read on Carmen's face that she knew. Once you've been a junkie, you gain a sixth sense for when other people are high. And 99 percent of the time, you're right. I did my best to stay alert and make jokes and follow the conversation and not nod out. I went to the kitchen for water and Carmen followed me.

"Hey, you okay?" she asked.

"Yeah, I'm good. Why?"

She glanced down and then back at me, looking me directly in the eye. "Are you high right now?"

"What? No. Are you serious?"

"Yeah, I'm serious."

"Well, no. I'm not high. I am tired, though."

"Okay, if you say so," she said and walked out of the kitchen.

I could feel the heat around my neck and ears, the familiar discomfort of lying. And it made me angry at her that she confronted me.

Over the next several months, Diana and I stopped and started using both together and separately multiple times. I'd use for a few weeks, get strung out, kick, stay clean for a few weeks, and then start all over again. I had some backward logic that stopping and starting and trying to control it made it less bad, made it only pretty bad.

But the problem was that Carmen wasn't the only one who

noticed. Pete confronted me. Alex confronted me. Carmen confronted me more than once. I lied to all of them and they didn't believe me, and I didn't care, or at least that's what I said to them. I started avoiding these people who cared about me.

In May, Michael called me. He was living with his girlfriend, the one he'd left me for. We made small talk and caught up on what we'd been doing. I left out my string of relapses.

"I miss you," he said.

"You do?"

"Yeah. I made a mistake."

"Yeah, well…okay."

"Can I see you?"

Every part of my body wanted to say no, knew that it was a bad idea. But another word came out of my mouth. "Okay."

Michael and I started spending time together, as friends at first. But by midsummer we were having an affair. I felt like I was back in the same position I'd put myself in with Vincent. The exception was Michael swore to me it was "mostly over" with his girlfriend, that they were living together while she got her finances in order and that was it. I knew I was being lied to, even though I told him I believed him. The conflict between what Michael told me and what my gut knew burned inside me, and I couldn't contain it.

In October, I was using regularly again. By the time Michael's girlfriend finally moved out at the end of the month, I tried to cut back on my heroin use, but there was always an excuse to keep me going. *Tomorrow, I'll stop tomorrow.* I was barely speaking to Carmen, which was challenging since we worked together. Pete was frequently out of town for work. I avoided Alex, sneaking in and out of my own house at times he wasn't there.

Michael, the person I saw most often, was finally catching on. By early November, he confronted me, or rather he caught me, and we broke up. He'd been suspicious and looked in my purse, finding my stash. We still spent my birthday together a couple of weeks later. He wanted me to get clean and I lied and told him I'd detoxed.

The week after Thanksgiving, I drove to meet my mom and her friend Cindy for a late lunch.

"You look a little puffy."

That's how it started. My mom touched my face, over pasta at Il Fornaio in Old Town Pasadena. The two leggy blondes across from me waited for a response.

"Puffy?"

"Have you been crying?"

I hadn't, though things weren't great. I didn't tell her that Michael and I had broken up again. I didn't tell her that I'd been dabbling with heroin again, off and on, and increasingly more on, and I was strung out. And I didn't tell her how challenging it was for me to get out of bed that morning, that my will to live had also been waning.

"No, I'm just PMS-ing. My period is a couple days late."

"Oh. Is there a chance you could be pregnant?" she asked.

"No," I said as I shook my head. "I mean, I don't think so."

The truth was I'd gone off the pill again and the last time I went off the pill was when I was with Jack. I *did* get pregnant then, and the abortion set off what was arguably the worst relapse of my life. Tuning out of the conversation, I sat there, scanning my memory for the exact date of my last period. I could tell by the excited chatter of my mom and Cindy that they were feeling good from their pinot grigio.

Cindy pulled out her cell phone and made a call. I excused myself to go to the bathroom. Maybe I'd get lucky; maybe I'd see signs of my period on the toilet paper, blood drops like tea leaves spelling out a fortune.

There was no such luck. I looked in the mirror while I washed my hands. *I do look a little puffy.* My short dark hair framed my thin but puffy face. I had bags under my eyes, and my pale olive skin was looking a little greenish again. Returning to the table, the two of them seemed excited about something. They were two peas in a pod, both tall and slim and a touch glamorous in that blonde and golden way I could never be. My mom's expression changed as she watched me approach the table.

"Erin, your breasts look huge."

This is something I'd *never* heard. I looked down at my chest as I sat down. *My boobs are puffy, too.*

"So," said Cindy, "we called Nordstrom at The Grove, and they have the new Marc Jacobs bags in, and they're holding them for us."

"I'll get you one as an early Christmas present," my mom chimed in.

I smiled, still contemplating my puffy-possibly-pregnant state.

"Let's get a pregnancy test, too, just so we know," my mom said, as if it were the most casual thing in the world.

Cindy nodded her head. These ladies were having way too much fun while I contemplated the horrifying possibility of another unwanted pregnancy. I touched my puffy face like I was testing it for a sign of something. My hands smelled like garlic, and it made my stomach turn.

"Don't touch your face, Erin. You'll break out," my mom said.

We drove on the 134 Freeway, then along Forest Lawn Drive and into Hollywood.

"Rite Aid!" Cindy said, pointing to the corner. "We can grab a pregnancy test."

"Now?" I asked.

Neither one of them answered, and my mom turned into the parking lot of Rite Aid, practically pushing me out the door. This was not the first time I'd bought a pregnancy test at this Rite Aid. The last time I'd gone in the middle of the night while Jack slept on my couch.

Francine Dancer sadly was not there, and it was too early for any sex workers. The sun was just setting. Echoing what I did the last time, I bought a test, some tampons and condoms, and

York Peppermint Patties. We arrived at The Grove, and my mom and Cindy insisted that I take the test, there, in the bathroom of Nordstrom.

The women's bathroom was nicer than your average public restroom, complete with a lounge, sporting gray velvet sofas, soft lighting, a long vanity, and large bathroom stalls. We were the only ones there. While Cindy touched up her makeup in the lounge, my mother waited impatiently outside the bathroom stall.

My hands shook as I tore open the box. I opened the foil wrapper and shut my eyes, trying to pee.

"Did you do it?"

"Mom, stop talking."

I wasn't exactly high, but I'd smoked heroin before meeting up with my mom and Cindy. There was enough in my system that I was what I like to call heroin pee shy. To remedy this, I did multiplication tables in my head. I don't know why this odd distraction worked, but it usually did. I'm sure there's a scientist somewhere who can explain it.

I managed to take the test without dousing my hand in urine. I laid the test down on a piece of toilet paper on top of the metal toilet paper holder. I had a bad metallic taste in my mouth. The taste was familiar. I had it the last time I was pregnant—like I'd been sucking on pennies.

My life, once more, felt like it was on repeat. Two years since the pregnancy and the abortion and Jack and the crack, and here I was, possibly pregnant again, chipping away, trying not to get strung out.

"Well?" my mom asked.

I picked up the test. There were two lines.

"Mom." I burst out of the stall, trembling, and showed her the test.

"Oh my God, oh my God, I'm so excited," she said, grabbing me by the shoulders.

"I need to sit down," I said, aware of the black dots floating in front of me. I was about to faint.

"Okay, sit down, honey."

Mom tried to reel in her excitement. She knew I wasn't sure what I was going to do. She bought me a black "Stella" Marc Jacobs bag, and she and Cindy continued shopping.

In a daze, I went outside to have a cigarette and call Diana. The Grove was all lit up with shimmering little Christmas lights, an enormous Christmas tree, and a model of Santa Claus and his sled and reindeer hung up in the sky. The air was cool and damp and soothing, counteracting the roiling heat of panic that flushed my cheeks.

Diana appropriately freaked out when I told her.

"What are you gonna do?" she asked.

"I don't know. I don't know."

I didn't know. From the outside, the simple answer seemed to be that I should have an abortion. I was barely functioning as an adult; I was using again. What other answer could there be?

When I finally got home that night, I called Michael and told him I was pregnant.

"How do you know it's mine?" he asked.

"Are you kidding? I haven't slept with anyone else."

"Are you using?"

"No, I've been clean for like a week."

Lies.

"I gotta go. We need to talk about this tomorrow. I can't really process this," he said.

I went to my bathroom, turned the lights off, sat down on the cold floor, and smoked some heroin. After stepping outside for a cigarette on my porch, I walked down to the basement and opened the door to Pete's room. He was out of town, working on a film. *It smells like him in here.* I walked over to the boom box on the shelf and looked through the small stacks of CDs. I pulled out *Radio Ethiopia* and put it in the CD player, flipping through to my favorite song. I lay down on his bed and looked at the photographs he had taped on the wall—photos he had taken on another trip. I curled up on his bed and listened to Patti Smith sing "Pissing in a River" and cried. *What am I gonna do? How did I get here? Again.*

I'd fallen asleep or nodded out in Pete's bed and dreamed about my corpse baby, which I hadn't done in a long while. *Is it a sign? I can't have this baby. Maybe I can? Maybe I'm supposed to? I have to get clean.*

For the next two weeks, I debated with myself, I discussed with Diana and Michael and my mom. My mom told my dad. But no one had all the information. Diana was the only one who knew I was using.

I drove to Michael's on a chilly December morning, pulled into his garage, and took a deep breath. I walked into the courtyard behind his house and looked up at the enormous old banyan tree that cradled the sky above the large gray house. I pushed open the French doors to Michael's bedroom. He was in bed still, playing guitar.

"Hey," he said.

I swallowed, took a breath, and said, "I'm going to have this baby."

He continued playing guitar and didn't say anything for a while. I stood in the doorway, looking down at my dark green Converses.

"You promise me you're not using, that you won't use?" he asked.

"I promise."

I felt like I was going to pass out.

Later that week, Michael and I drove into the Valley. My dad was in town, and my parents wanted to talk to us about "our plans." We were meeting them at Olga and Ken's house. As I drove, Michael was thinking out loud about logistics—would we live together and which house would we live in. I listened with a knot in my stomach.

As we drove up the narrow winding road to the house, Michael suddenly said, "Pull over. Stop the car."

I did and said, "What? What's wrong?"

Michael got out of the car and walked around to the driver's side, tapping on the window. I rolled it down. His eyes, the color of sea glass, were gleaming beneath the brim of his narrow gray tartan hat.

He started laughing. "It smells like horse shit."

"Yeah, because there are horses right there," I said, pointing to the paddock across the street.

He took my hand and said, "Let's get married."

"What?"

"Let's get married. Fuck it. Let's give it a shot."

"You don't have to marry me. I didn't ask… That's not why I want to have the baby."

"I know, but let's do it. Let's try to make it work."

I was stunned.

"Well?"

"Okay," I said.

"Okay?"

"Yes, let's give it a shot."

My head swam. I knew that it was a mistake. I had been addicted to Michael. I had wanted him to want me, to love me, but I knew that what I felt for him wasn't love; it was a need to be desired. I pushed that aside and tried to convince myself that it was love; it was destiny. I held hope that maybe this would turn me around. *Maybe he's just what I need. Maybe he can save me.* The first thing I had to do was get clean again.

What have I done?

CHAPTER 23
Like a Happened Balloon
April 2003

And you float all around
like a happened balloon.
> —Anne Sexton, "Admonitions to a Special Person"

"Erin, could you walk a little faster please."

I glared at my mom as I walked across her perfectly green lawn toward the driveway, and slowed my gait.

"Erin!"

I started running. I ran right past her, onto the buckled sidewalk, down the wide street flanked by picture-perfect houses set back from the road by large swaths of green grass. I ran down the hill, tears rolling down my cheeks and floating off my face with the breeze made from running. I ran down Meridian Street toward Mission all the way to the South Pasadena Public Library. I sat on a bench and put my hands over my bump, the bump that housed the tiny baby growing inside me that I didn't yet feel emotionally connected to, and I tried to slow my breath down, to stop myself from hyperventilating.

Earlier that day, my mom and I had been at my house in Echo
Park, packing up my things. I felt frustrated with her—not with
her, with myself, but the frustration had nowhere else to go. I'd
thrown my phone and broken it. We'd gone back to her house
for lunch and to get more boxes, and then I snapped at her comment about my slow walking.

Michael and I had married in February. Our marriage was
off to an awful start. When he'd discovered I was still using, he
stuck by me and went through with the wedding, but he held
the drug use over my head like a guillotine.

Diana had helped me find a doctor who would detox me
with buprenorphine. All the other doctors wanted me to go on
methadone, and I'd refused. I didn't want my baby to be born
addicted to anything. Over the course of seven days, I detoxed
with the help of the meds. A few weeks later, Diana did the
same. She was just about the only person I was still speaking to;
I'd pushed everyone away. I didn't invite Carmen or Alex or
Pete to the wedding. Lila and I stopped speaking. CeCe and I
stopped talking. And I'd been ghosting most everyone else because I was so ashamed.

It was a new level of contempt I felt for myself. I'd crossed yet
another line I had never imagined crossing. I'd used heroin while
pregnant. It was one thing when I was harming myself. Now I
had endangered my unborn child. The stigma of that felt overwhelming and I knew everyone knew, or they suspected. Even
once I'd detoxed, the residue of what I'd done haunted me, and
I felt like I couldn't face the people who knew, people I loved.

For our honeymoon, we went to Maui and stayed at the Ritz-
Carlton. Michael and I hiked to see waterfalls, we ate in the
moonlight overlooking the ocean, we went snorkeling, but the
reality of our marriage crept up like quicksand. I hated the way
he ate. He controlled his food to the extent that all he ate was
salad, seaweed, and avocado. His resentment at me for having

used while pregnant surged to the surface over dinner, at the beach, when we were alone in our room. Neither of us wanted to be there. By there, I mean with each other, pretending to be a happy newlywed couple. But I was desperate to get my life back on track, any track.

When we returned from Maui, I didn't want to move into Michael's house—it was gloomy and in disrepair. My house in Echo Park wasn't fit for a baby. The plan was to sell my place, look for something new, and have Michael keep his house to be used as a recording studio. In the time that I'd known him, his career, which had once been on fire, was shaky. He'd borrowed money from my parents to upgrade his studio.

One afternoon, shortly after Maui, I grabbed my laptop from Michael's nightstand and settled myself on his bed to look at some houses. A breeze came in from the courtyard, through the open French doors, the billowy pale blue curtains rising and falling. Some guys were working upstairs repairing the deck and listening to "Clocks" by Coldplay, which seemed to always be on the radio at the time.

When I opened my laptop, I saw that Michael had left his Hotmail open and the email staring back at me was from June, one of his ex-girlfriends. The first sentence I read was I'm not having the abortion.

A rush of adrenaline rose in my chest, and my mouth got watery as if I was going to throw up. As I read on through their email exchange, my ears began to ring, and I had trouble breathing.

She said, If you can do this with Erin, you can do this with me.

He said, The only reason I'm doing this with Erin is because her parents have money. I don't love her.

I slammed my computer shut and forced myself to concentrate on breathing. I wanted a cigarette or heroin or a knife. It felt impossible to sit there stewing in the myriad of things I was feeling, but I had to. The alternative was running back to heroin. As much as I wanted to escape, I didn't want that baby to be born addicted and I'd come this far. I dug deep and found the will to stay, to sit, to not exit. Michael popped his head in a few minutes later.

"I'm running to Whole Foods. Do you need anything?"

"We need to talk," I said.

"Now?"

"Yeah, now."

I opened my laptop and pushed it across the bed toward him.

He bent down and squinted at the screen and said, "So, you're reading my fucking email now?"

"You left it open. On my computer."

"Yeah, well, congratulations, junior detective."

"What?"

"What do you need to talk about?" he asked.

"Um, the fact that June is pregnant. That you've been cheating on me, again, this whole time. That you don't love me. That you're using me."

"You know, Erin, you have no fucking room to say a fucking word to me about anything. You want me to call your dad and tell him his little princess was still doing heroin until I stepped in? That you kept using after you found out you were pregnant? You will lose this baby so fast. You think a court is gonna look kindly on a junkie mom who cared more about heroin than her unborn child?"

I breathed in and out rapidly, and hot, angry, scared tears had nowhere to go but down my face. "I'm clean, Michael."

"Yeah, now, thanks to me. Do you know how demoralizing and lonely it was to deal with this shit without anyone to talk to about it? June was there for me."

"But you must have gotten her pregnant before you found out I was still using."

"Oh, you don't know anything," he said, and he slammed the French door behind him on the way out.

When he came back a few hours later, he was repentant. He told me that June did end up having an abortion, that he loved me, and that he wanted to make it work.

In the weeks that followed, I spent most nights at my mom's. No one asked me why I wasn't staying at my own house or with my husband. When Michael and I spent time together, it was tense, and we spoke about practical matters like strollers or ultrasounds or a new house that came on the market. Physical intimacy between the two of us stopped altogether. We both had so much resentment toward each other. I resented him for cheating and lying, and he resented me for using and lying.

By April, when I was moving my things into storage, I felt lost and angry and scared most of the time. And I feared that I'd never be able to do it—be a mom, stay clean, stay sane. I read a lot of Sylvia Plath and Anne Sexton. I felt haunted by their words, by their lives. We were all Scorpios; we were all a little intense. Would I end up like they did, dying by suicide? Would I leave that legacy for this kid?

I was supposed to be happy and glowing and in love with my unborn child and my new husband. But most days, I still fantasized about killing myself. This kid wasn't even here yet, and I was already failing miserably. What if I relapsed again?

I had $5 in the pocket of my bubble gum–pink maternity trench coat. The bright pink was an odd color choice for me, one that seemed to scream I was trying to be anything other than who I had been before. It was starting to cool off, the late-afternoon sky painted with streaks of orange and pink, and I could smell the tamales from the Thursday evening farmers market. I walked toward the food stalls, my $5 in hand, my stomach rumbling.

"Erin?"

I heard a familiar voice behind me and spun around. It was Mary—my old sponsor and good friend—and her six-year-old daughter.

"Hi. Oh my gosh, I thought you'd already moved," I said as we hugged.

"No, next week."

Mary and her daughter were moving back East to Connecticut. They were going to move in with her mom while she went to design school in Manhattan.

We walked through the farmers market and talked about her move and the fight with my mom and how I'd broken my phone.

"You have to come visit," she said before they left.

"I will!"

I bought kettle corn and lemonade with my $5 and walked to a pay phone where I called my mom, collect.

"Mom, can you come get me?"

I walked back to the benches in front of the library and sat down, waiting for my mom. She pulled up ten minutes later in her black Mercedes sedan and smiled when she saw me. When I got in the car, she burst out laughing.

"What's so funny?" I said, laughing with her.

"You just looked pitiful sitting there with your little baby bump and your bag of popcorn and lemonade."

It was funny. I felt like the petulant child who'd run away from home and called her mommy to pick her up from the park an hour later. It was a pretty accurate picture.

We were both consumed by giggles.

"I'm sorry, Mom."

"It's okay. You're hormonal. I love you."

At the end of April, Michael and I had a big fight. We'd met Diana for dinner at The Newsroom on Robertson. I can't remember how the fight started, but at some point he said, "You know, your parents and I had a long talk about what we're going to do when you relapse again."

Diana tried to mediate. "Michael, that's not very helpful."

"Well, we all know it's inevitable."

"Fuck you," I said.

We sat in silence, punctuated by Diana's attempts at small talk.

When we got back to Michael's house, I said, "My dad is in town this weekend. I'm gonna go back East with him for a while."

"I think that's a great idea."

I spent about a month back East. It was a relief being there, away from Michael. I drove down to Connecticut and spent time with Mary, too. We drove around listening to The White Stripes and Eminem. We stayed up late at night talking like teenagers. We had a magical night out in the city, seeing The Flaming Lips play and barhopping with an actor friend. I felt more like myself than I had in a long time.

More important, Mary was the only friend I had who was a mother. We talked about motherhood and my fears about staying clean and dealing with Michael.

"I don't feel connected to this baby at all. Like, what if I feel nothing when it's born. What if I can't stay clean?"

"You will."

"I don't know... You know my parents and Michael are convinced I won't be able to do it. I feel like they're all taking bets on when I'm gonna relapse."

Mary took my hand and looked at me with shiny, loving eyes, and said, "I am 100 percent sure you can do this, Erin. I believe it with all my heart."

For the first time, I felt like maybe I could do this. Maybe I could be an okay mom to this baby. I needed those words of encouragement.

When I got back to LA, my house sold. Michael and I were cordial with each other, but I was still spending most nights away.

In those last few months of pregnancy, I became closer to my friend Danica whom I'd met through Michael and had been friends with for a couple years. A curvy blonde with a quick wit who seemingly knew everyone in Hollywood, she always wore lipstick, even with pajamas. Danica was a little older than me, had many years of sobriety under her belt, and had known Michael since they were teenagers. She was wonderful at helping me deal with Michael and diffuse some of the animosity between us. I felt safe with Danica; she was like a big sister to me. My third trimester was largely spent with her—going to the movies, eating Indian takeout, watching reality shows in bed. Much as Mary had, Danica was like a guide helping me find myself again, helping me believe I could be a mom and stay sober.

By July, it was clear I wasn't going to find a new house before the baby came. The housing market in LA in 2003 was on a high, and I'd been outbid on several homes. I took an apartment at The Palazzo across from The Grove, the site of my public restroom pregnancy test months prior. It was a new building, close to Michael's house, and I didn't have to lock into a long lease. We moved in on July 15, a few weeks from my due date, and my mom and I scrambled to get things set up.

As the last few days of July crawled by, I started having contractions. I went to the hospital twice. I was under two centimeters dilated, and it wasn't progressing. But I was in prodromal labor. Ready or not, this was happening.

CHAPTER 24

Atticus

Cedars Sinai Hospital
August 1, 2003

"All right, honey, we're going to start the Pitocin drip," said Shelly, the labor and delivery nurse who looked like Doris Day.

Shifting, anxious, and uncomfortable, swollen from nine months of pregnancy, I smiled at her. My mom was on the phone, and she smiled back at me from the corner of the small room. Earlier that morning, after being in early labor for days, my mom drove me to the obstetrician's office. He suggested we induce. I was 100 percent sure he'd made this call because it was Friday and he didn't want to be interrupted over the weekend. I was also 100 percent sure that I *wanted* to be induced. My pregnancy had been challenging for me in every way possible—physically of course, but emotionally, mentally, spiritually, and psychically as well.

"We're going to get you into a *real* labor and delivery room as soon as possible, sweetie. This is the busiest day we've had this year."

Again, shifting, anxious, and uncomfortable, I smiled. The nurse hummed loudly as she exited the room. I wished it didn't smell like Band-Aids and Betadine; the smells reminded me of detoxing and rehabs. I began to feel a little clammy and reminded myself to breathe.

While we waited for the Pitocin to take effect, that small room, no bigger than a walk-in closet, began to fill up. My dad arrived. Olga and Ken and their daughter, Sara, came. Michael's brother and mother, who felt like strangers to me, and his mother's random business associate arrived.

Everyone crowded around me, patting my arm, making jokes. I could sense their apprehension over how I was going to handle this, how I was going to be a mother to this baby boy. Or at least that was how I read the room. *They're all waiting for me to go crazy again.*

One person wasn't there yet—Michael. I asked my mom for my phone and called him. He didn't answer. I wasn't surprised; it was typical of these past nine months. Still, no matter what he'd done or said, I felt guilty. I was the one who'd used drugs while I was pregnant. I was the one who lied and hid it and endangered our baby. He had the upper hand, and I felt like he deserved it—no matter how often he lied to me and cheated on me.

I thought about Michael as my contractions started to kick in, the Pitocin doing its job. Getting married, going through with our shotgun wedding, had been a huge mistake. Experiencing yet another moment that Michael failed to support me as a partner, I questioned what I saw in Michael in the first place. A stronger contraction made me wince.

"Erin, are you okay?" my mom asked, noticing I'd blanched and was sweating.

"I think the Pitocin is working."

A different nurse came in—Naomi. Her beautiful accent made me think she was from an island.

"How are you doing, Erin?" She spoke loudly, slowly, like a preschool teacher.

"Uh, I'm okay. I think the Pitocin is working."

"Good! You tell me how strong your contractions are," she said, pointing to a pain measurement scale on the wall.

I pointed to face 1–2, which read, "Hurts just a little bit."

"Okay, then, I'll be back. I'm gonna check on your L&D room."

My phone started ringing, but I couldn't reach it. "Mom, could you?"

She handed me the phone. It was Michael.

"Heyyyyyy. I'm on my way, but I got in a little car accident."

"What? In my car?" I asked, not inquiring if he was okay.

"Yeah, but don't worry, the woman's cool. So, I'm, like, around the corner. My mom might get there before I do."

"She's already here," I seethed. "Bye."

"Is he on his way?" asked Mom.

"He got in a freaking car accident."

"In your car?" my dad asked.

"Yes."

My parents exchanged a glance. Even though they were both remarried, had been separated for more than twenty years and divorced for more than a decade, they still possessed the ability to communicate via glances. I admired it. I felt like I'd spent my entire life waiting for an invitation, a way into their secret language.

Michael's mom and brother and random business associate came back in to check on me.

"Wow, you're huge," said Michael's brother.

I nodded and smiled and thought, *No shit, asshole.* There were suddenly eight people in my walk-in closet, and I was starting to feel claustrophobic. My contractions were getting stronger. Naomi, the nurse, came back in and immediately recognized the panic on my face.

"All right, I need everyone to leave the room for a while," she said, guiding them out the door with hands on their backs.

Everyone left except for my mother.

"You, too, Mommy," Naomi said, glancing at my mom.

"I'll be right outside," my mom said as she exited.

Apparently, Naomi was also privy to my parents' secret language of glances. This time, when she pointed at the pain chart, I told her I was a 3–4, the one that read, "Hurts a little more." She checked my cervix.

"You're only about four centimeters. That's good. Okay, I'll be back."

For a brief moment, I was left alone in the room, staring at "hurts a little more," wondering if I'd be able to handle this when I got to 9–10.

Michael appeared in the doorway, with a large salad bowl and fork. *A fucking salad bowl—are you kidding me?* He stood there, chewing, with seaweed in his teeth. I could smell him from the door—olive oil, dulse seaweed, avocado, and paprika. This didn't mix well with the Band-Aids and Betadine.

"You brought a salad with you?"

"Yeah," he laughed. "I hadn't eaten. That's what took me a while. I had to go to Whole Foods, and then go home and make it," he said while eating, exposing all the ingredients.

"So, what happened?"

"I just told you."

"No, with the car accident."

"Oh. Well, I was at a red light on Third Street, like two blocks from Cedars, and I took a bite of my salad. The light turned green, so I started to go, and then the woman in front of me braked and I rear-ended her. But it's seriously no big deal. There's hardly a scratch on your car."

"And her car?"

"She has a little damage but hardly anything. I gave her your information."

"Gee, thanks."

I despised this man. I despised this man, and I was about to give birth to his baby. *Maybe I will move back to France. Maybe my mom should raise the baby.* My thoughts spiraled for a moment, focusing in on all the ways I felt trapped. A contraction knocked them away again. *I can do this.* I gritted my teeth through the gripping pain. Michael smiled at me again with his seaweed teeth. My parents walked back in. My stepdad was with them. He's a good guy. Not much of a talker, but he always showed up. I could hear the voices of the others in the hallway.

"Maybe you should go check on your mom," I said to Michael.

He nodded and smiled and left the room. My mom sat on the edge of the bed. My dad's best friend, Ken, came in again with Sara. Growing up as only children, Sara felt like a sister to me and I was happy to see her face right then. Michael came back and told us that his mom and company were going to Orso for dinner. I suggested he go with them and he agreed, said he'd go for a little while. *Relief.*

"Hello!" a voice called from the hallway, as an arm appeared, pushing a unicorn on a stick into the room.

"Hello?"

It was Danica, the lifesaver of a friend for my third trimester. She had been the one who took me to Apple Pan numerous times for pie, who danced with me, who ate breakfast with me at 1:00 a.m. at Pacific Dining Car while making a list of baby names, who supplied me with all the healthy distractions at her disposal, and who let me stay countless nights at her apartment while I avoided Michael.

"Hi! I brought you a whole chocolate cream pie from Marie Callender's and a pony—well, a unicorn."

"I am so happy to see you." And I meant it.

Another contraction came on strong, just as Naomi walked in. "Oh, you've got more visitors."

"I brought her pie and a pony-corn," said Danica.

"She can't have the pie."

"Oh, that's fine," I said. "Why don't you take it?"

Naomi laughed and took the pie, thanking me. She let me keep the pony/unicorn and pointed to the chart.

"Five–six, 'hurts even more,'" I said.

"Okay, I'm going to be back in ten minutes to check on you."

Danica hugged me goodbye. Everyone else was out in the hallway or the cafeteria—everyone but my mom. I had lost count of how many visitors I had in and out of that tiny room in the past two hours. Another contraction hit me, and I looked at 7–8, "hurts a whole lot," knowing this was all getting very real.

"Mom, I don't know if I can do this."

My mom took my hand and tried to assure me that everything was going to be "just fine." But she looked worried. She knew that I didn't mean getting through that night. She left to find Naomi. Michael was not back yet, and if I could have left—left that body, left that room—run away, let everything go behind me, I would have. Right then, at that moment, I would have. But the contractions had me immobilized.

I was not breathing properly and couldn't remember anything from my childbirth class the month before. Michael wouldn't have been a help if he had been there. He'd only attended half of the classes with me. One night he went to a Nick Cave concert. One night he said he forgot because he was caught up with work in the studio. Both times I'd wondered if he was really with June.

My mom returned with Naomi.

"Naomi, I'm at 7–8," I said.

"Okay, Erin, I'm going to get Dr. Fitz."

Lying there, waiting, I held my mom's hand, and I thought about the fact that I picked Dr. Fitz out of a book that my crappy HMO COBRA insurance provided. I chose him because I liked his name and his office was by the good bagel place in Beverly Hills.

"How are we doing?" Dr. Fitz asked as he waltzed in. "Do you want an epidural? Now's the time."

He had me at *epi.*

"We have to break your water before we put the catheter in."

I insisted on peeing before the catheter, which made no sense but they let me do it anyway. The bathroom in my walk-in closet room was the size of an airplane bathroom. It's a miracle I didn't pee on the floor. When I waddled back into my walk-in closet, Michael had returned, and Dr. Fitz was waiting with the anesthesiologist and a giant hook. I might have stopped breathing.

Lying back down on the bed, I watched Michael's eyes widen as Dr. Fitz stuck the giant hook inside me. *Holy shit.* And then my water broke. It was a relief, a release of pressure. I continued watching Michael's face—displaying a mix of horror and fascination—as Dr. Fitz threaded that catheter right up in me. The anesthesiologist had me lie on my side, and I felt pressure and a sharp spike of pain as he inserted a massive needle into the base of my spine. I couldn't see Michael's face, but I heard him when he said, "OH SHIT."

And then, I got some relief. Dr. Fitz told me I was about six centimeters dilated and it would be a few more hours. I was so fucking grateful to not be in pain. I shut my eyes and slept for a few minutes. When I opened my eyes, about twenty-five minutes after the epidural, I noticed I was beginning to feel my contractions again.

"Can you get Naomi?" I asked Michael.

It took him an eternity because everything Michael did always took forever—from making a salad to fetching a nurse—like he was moving through life in slow motion. By the time he returned with her, I was in more pain than I was before the epidural.

"I'm at 9–10, 9–10!"

Naomi looked at me suspiciously, like she didn't believe me. Nine-ten is "hurts as much as you can imagine, you don't have to be crying to feel this bad." But when she looked at the monitor, she saw that I was not breathing well. The baby's heart rate was dropping, and we were not getting enough oxygen. She put an oxygen mask on me and checked my cervix.

"Well, I know why you're hurting. You are ten centimeters, Erin. Wow. You dilated four centimeters in less than thirty minutes."

Hooray for Pitocin. I guess this is why people tell you not to induce.

Naomi ran out and returned with the anesthesiologist, who removed the epidural. "We are trying to get you an L&D room, okay? Whatever you do, don't push."

"Don't push?"

It was easier said than done because I could feel the pressure of that tiny, tiny human who was so eager to emerge.

"Mom? I don't know if I can do this."

This time she exchanged a glance with Michael. I tried to decipher what the glance meant. *Maybe they all don't know if I can do this. How the fuck did I get here?*

After an excruciating half hour, they quickly, finally wheeled me into a labor and delivery room. I was hoisted onto a new bed, and they got my wobbly legs up into stirrups. Unbeknownst to me, my mom stood in the corner. Michael and Naomi each took a leg and coached me to push.

After twenty minutes of pushing, shortly after 1:00 a.m. on August 2, 2003, I gave birth to Atticus. I waited those eternal ten seconds to hear him cry out.

"You have a healthy baby boy," Naomi said, and she placed him on my chest. We looked into each other's eyes, Atticus and I. *Oh, it's you*, I thought. I knew him. I knew this soul in the body of a baby. I'd been waiting for him for a lifetime.

After years of feeling lost at sea, everything came together and made sense in that very moment. His birth was a miracle, a turning point. A switch flipped. *I love him more than I hate myself. I love him more than I hate myself.*

I knew I would never use drugs again, and I didn't. This sounds overly simple. Maybe it is. Maybe I got lucky. Maybe I won the lottery. There would be work to come—spiritual, emotional, mental, cognitive work to do—but things would never be the same again. He saved my life.

Mom walked over to me as I held this little being, and she saw the shift in my eyes. She put her hand on my heart.

"I hope you're not mad. I was in the room and they didn't kick me out."

I looked at her with tears streaming down my cheeks and said, "I don't care, Mom. Look at him. I didn't know how it would feel. I didn't think I could love him. I love him. I love him. I didn't think I could love like this."

"I know, honey, I know. He's your guardian angel."

CHAPTER 25
Long Time Sun
August 2003–2005

When we brought Atticus home from the hospital, I felt determined—both to be a good mom to this boy and to make my marriage work. I desperately didn't want Atticus to be a child of divorce like I was. Before we left the hospital, I grabbed Michael's hand and said, "We can do this, right? We can start over and make this marriage work?"

He paused for a moment. It was a mere moment but it hung in the air like a thousand moments. His pale eyes shifted from blue to green in the light.

"Yeah. Yeah, I think we can make it work."

"No more lies. No more cheating. No more drugs."

He hugged me in response.

When we got home, neighbors were moving into the apartment below. There were still very few occupied apartments in the brand-new building. Michael and I were out on our balcony with Atticus, in the shade, taking in the warm air of the late afternoon, listening to the fountains bubble away in the courtyard when a voice called up. I bounced up and down on my heels as Atticus fussed.

"Is that a baby I hear up there?"

Michael leaned over the edge and introduced himself to Bea, the woman downstairs. I didn't see her, but her voice was remarkably sunny. A few weeks later, I ran into her in the parking garage, on my way home from the pediatrician with Atticus. A very tall, very thin, smiling blonde woman with glasses introduced herself.

"Hi! I'm Bea. I think I met your husband. We live below you."

She was so friendly and bright, I liked her instantly. Bea and her husband, Dale, had moved in while they were renovating an old fixer-upper. Dale was a musician and the world's best home cook, and Bea was a stay-at-home mom. They had three kids: two from his first marriage and an eighteen-month-old boy they'd adopted named Delaney. Bea and Dale and their family were everything I wished my little family with Michael could be. They were warm and generous and a team.

I was woozy—exhausted from several days of little sleep and the uncharted territory of motherhood. I was equally intoxicated by what it was like loving another being with absolute devotion. I needed grounding. Michael's help was limited. Bea and Dale became my family. I ate dinner with them more often than not. They taught me how to cook and take care of my home, how to get Atticus on a schedule, and how to be a parent. I don't know how I would have survived those early months had I not met them.

Most nights, Michael was at the studio and would come home at four or five in the morning, often smelling of freesia. I knew he was cheating on me. I knew he wouldn't keep his promise.

When Atticus was about a month old, I was up with him at 3:00 a.m. He was colicky, and I was sleep deprived. I'd called Michael over and over again. He didn't pick up. I finally put Atticus in my Volvo station wagon and drove the two minutes over to the studio. He wasn't there. It was all locked up. *He's with her.* I didn't know yet which her, but I knew there was *a her.*

As I drove around the block back to the apartment, I noticed two people sitting in a car. I slowed down and looked. It was Michael and June in June's car. In a blind rage, I stopped my car and tore the driver's side door open. June got out, and we fought—pulling each other's hair and shouting obscenities. Atticus screamed from the back of my car. Michael stood there and then yelled at me to stop—the baby needed me. I let go of June and got in my car and drove off with June screaming behind me, Atticus wailing in the back seat.

I got home and took Atticus to bed and nursed him. When Michael got back, Atticus was asleep next to me. Michael sat down on the bed and didn't say anything.

"You fucking lied to me. You promised you'd try. He's not even a month old." I started crying again, and I hated myself for it.

"You know, June is the only person that has been there for me through all this—when you were using and everything. I didn't want to let her down. But it's over now."

I wanted to believe him.

"I love you, and I want us to be a family," I said. Even as the words came out of my mouth, I knew they weren't entirely true. I felt like I was trying to convince myself that I loved him. But I didn't. My desire for stability, of what I thought a family should look like argued otherwise.

"You won't find anyone else who would put up with you," he said.

For months after this fight, we were caught in a dysfunctional cycle. I knew he was cheating; I'd confront him, and he'd say I was imagining things and acting crazy, and I'd stuff it away. Without heroin, without self-harm, without sex, without all the old coping mechanisms I'd had, I struggled with anxiety and depression. But I had to push forward. I had to for Atticus, even in the moments when I didn't think I could.

I reverted back to an even older coping mechanism I'd had as a small child—hold my breath, count, disconnect from my body. I spent empty hours online, on eBay, buying vintage toys for Atticus that I'd had as a kid. I let myself sit in the hostility I had toward Michael. That hostility slowly became armor. These were not the healthiest or most effective strategies for what I was going through, but they were better than self-harm. They were better than relapsing. Like they teach you in recovery groups, I focused on getting through one day at a time, one hour at a time, sometimes one minute at a time.

I kept myself busy with looking at houses for sale, taking care of Atticus, and spending time with Bea. When Dale went on tour, Bea and I were like sister wives—sharing kid duty, making dinner together, and I tried to ignore how much my hatred of Michael was growing. Other times I leaned right into it.

One Sunday afternoon in January 2004, I had just come out of the shower and could hear that Michael was talking on the house phone. Atticus was napping on our bed. I felt that familiar intuition in my gut. *Things have been going better. He made resolutions. We've been getting along. But...something is off.* When I came out of the bathroom, he was hanging up. He went and put the phone back on the charging station in the living room.

"I'm gonna take a shower," he said.

I nodded. My stomach clenched. I knew. I picked up the phone and hit Redial.

"Hello," a female voice answered.

"Who is this?" I asked.

"Who is this?" she snapped back.

"June?"

"Erin?"

I began to cry. "He promised me. He promised me it was over with you," I said.

"I'm sorry, Erin. I wouldn't have gotten back together with him. He told me it was over with you guys."

"How long?" I asked.

"What?"

"How long this time?"

Silence.

"Months?"

"Yes," she replied. "Look, this is fucked up. I think we need to sit Michael down and ask him what he wants to do."

When Michael got out of the shower, I was still on the phone with June, sitting on the bed in a towel.

"What are you doing?" he asked. "Why aren't you dressed?"

"I know."

"What?"

"I'm talking to June."

He wouldn't respond. I followed him around the room as he got dressed and ignored me. I screamed at him, June listening from the other end of the phone.

He walked out the door, and I chased after him in my towel like a madwoman. The door slammed behind me, and I realized I had just locked myself out in my towel and that Atticus was locked inside. June called his cell and got him to come back and unlock the door. He took off again.

"I'm coming over. He has to come back sometime," said June.

I called Bea. She and Dale had recently moved into their newly renovated home, about a ten-minute drive away. Through tears, I told her what was going on. I asked her if she could come get Atticus and take him to her house for a while. She did, just as June arrived.

June looked weary. Her long dark hair framed her pale narrow face, her blue eyes red from crying. "I'm really sorry, Erin." She hugged me. She smelled like freesia.

"You know what, June? This is Michael's fault, not yours."

I told her about finding the emails and how he held my drug use over my head. We drove to his studio. He wasn't there. We came back to the apartment and waited. An hour later, he finally came back.

"What the fuck…" he said when he walked in the door.

He sat down, and June and I took turns spelling out the lies he'd told us each. He sat there, mostly silent, playing with a hole in the knee of his blue corduroy pants.

"What is it you want?" asked June. "Because you can't go on like this with both of us."

He didn't respond.

"Do you even love me? Do you want this marriage to work?" I asked.

He looked at me and said, "How could I love you? You're a broken fucking dog."

"Michael, stop it," said June.

That moment, that searingly painful moment stands out for me as one of the cruelest things Michael ever said to me. It encapsulated all the fears I had about myself. *I am broken. I am ugly. I am unlovable. No one will ever love you.*

I went into the bedroom and sobbed, the kind of cries that start in the center of your gut and contract your entire body, spreading the shards of emotional pain to the edge of your skin. My cell phone rang. It was Bea. Atticus was crying. It had been hours since I'd nursed him.

"I have to go get Atticus," I said.

"Well, I'm done here. I'm done with you, Michael," June said. She touched my arm on her way out. "I hope you leave him. You don't deserve this."

I grabbed my keys and headed to the garage. Michael followed me, silent. On the drive, he finally spoke.

"Erin, I'm sorry. I didn't mean what I said. I want to be a family. I love Atticus more than anything in the world. But I don't think I want to be romantic with you. It's just dead for me."

I said nothing.

"Just remember who stood by you when you were pregnant and using heroin. Do you know what your parents would do if they knew? They'd take Atticus."

When we got to Bea and Dale's, they were just about to have dinner. Atticus was swollen with tears, in his little white T-shirt and baby denim overalls. I took him in my arms and he shuddered with relief. I nursed Atticus in the cozy Craftsman living room, all wood and subdued colors, while Michael stood awkwardly in the dining room and made small talk while they ate. It was clear Bea had filled in her family. They were stiff and silent in response.

Before we left, Bea pulled me aside and said, "Erin, don't put up with his shit. He's not going to change."

"But you don't understand," I said.

The next day, I walked down Third Street to the Golden Bridge—a Kundalini yoga center that was known for its pre- and postnatal classes. The owner, Gurmukh—a Sikh woman in flowing white linen who emanated healing energy—led the class. With a room of people, all mothers, we moved our bodies through yoga poses, our babies lying on the floor by our sides or crawling around from mat to mat.

Gurmukh's soothing voice was a salve. She didn't just teach yoga; she taught motherhood. She spoke about the fears and anxieties we might feel. She talked about connecting with the little souls roaming around the room. At the close of the class, she ended it, as I would come to learn all the classes there ended, by playing a song, "Long Time Sun." The song comes from the words of Yogi Bhajan, the yogi who brought Kundalini yoga to the United States.

I held six-month-old Atticus in my arms and cried tears of hope as a woman sang, "May the longtime sun shine upon you, all love surround you, and the pure light within you guide your way on."

My heart knew I was exactly where I was supposed to be. I felt like I was home with these women.

From that day on, I took Atticus to baby yoga at least twice a week. It became the closest thing to "church" I'd ever had. I began to discover a spiritual center inside me, one I didn't know existed. As I connected with that inner self and focused on self-care, for maybe the first time, I disconnected from Michael. I didn't need him. I didn't need to pretend the marriage was something it wasn't.

Still, I didn't walk away from the marriage, for Atticus.

Just before Atticus's birthday, we moved into a house, a classic white Colonial with black shutters that was around the corner from Bea and Dale's renovated home in an old mid-city neighborhood called Country Club Park. We went through the motions of domestic life as we set up house. We had separate bedrooms. We argued a lot. Michael continued to be with other women and threaten me with losing custody because of my past. As time wore on, I believed his threat less and less.

On a trip to Las Vegas, visiting Michael's family, I went out to breakfast with his sister Rita. She seemed distracted when we sat down and placed our order.

"Rita, are you okay?"

She pursed her lips and shut her eyes, flipping her long brown hair. She took a breath and said, "Michael is building a case against you."

"What?" I asked. I pulled my hands up from the blue Formica table, sticky with the maple syrup of pancakes past.

"He's telling everyone you're mentally unstable, maybe on drugs again. If I were you, Erin, I would get out. My brother said he wants to get custody of Atticus and collect child support."

The only way out is through.

"Erin? Did you hear me?"

"Yes, I hear you."

When we got home from that trip, I knew I needed to tell everyone everything—that I had used early on in my pregnancy. I was petrified of what they'd think of me, if it would bring up all the old shame I'd spent a long time running from. I hoped that it would do the opposite. I knew I had to disentangle myself from Michael, and from the shame.

At my mom's, I sat with her in the den, on the comfy brown leather couch while Atticus played with my old wooden blocks on the floor.

"Mom, I need to tell you something."

"What is it?"

I told her that I'd used in my first trimester, that I didn't stop immediately, that I had to detox with a doctor.

"Honey, I already know."

"You know?"

"Michael told your dad and me months ago."

"And you didn't say anything?"

"Well, he was trying to suggest that you may be using again, but we both can see that's not true."

I sat there, shocked. I shouldn't have been shocked. Michael's greatest defense mechanism was gaslighting people into what he wanted them to believe. Of course he would try this on my parents.

I told Bea and Dale. "I knew he was holding something over your head," Bea said when I told them.

I told Danica. Michael had already told her, too.

What amazed me was that no one believed him. Yes, they thought that I'd been on drugs in early pregnancy, but his assertion that I was using again—none of them bought it because I showed up, I cared for Atticus, I was acting like an adult, finally.

I didn't tell Michael that I knew what he'd been up to. Instead, I bided my time, preparing myself emotionally and building a support system. Atticus and I spent a lot of time at my mom's and we visited my dad back East frequently. We hung out with

Bea and Delaney all the time, especially when Dale was tour-
ing. We swam at their house almost every day, took the kids to
Disneyland with annual passes, went thrift store shopping, ate
at Joan's on Third, and went to the park. I'd made other friends
from yoga. I had a community of people to lean on. I'd made
the family I'd wanted so badly, without Michael.

By the fall of 2005, Bea and I decided to start a business
together—a clothing line. Atticus started preschool a few days a
week. And Michael was consumed by another affair that I again
ignored. One afternoon, I was cleaning up toys in the sunroom
when my cell phone rang. It was an old actor friend from New
York whom Mary and I had hung out with when I was pregnant.
We made small talk for a bit. I wondered why he was calling.

"So, the reason I called is that I wanted to know if you and
Michael are still together."

"Yeah, why?"

He waited for a moment on the phone. "Erin, he's in a relationship with Carla," he said, naming the woman I suspected
Michael had been seeing. "They're openly, publicly together. I
ran into them at a gallery opening last week."

"Oh. It doesn't surprise me."

"Can I ask you something?"

"Yeah."

"Why are you still with him?"

"I have no fucking idea."

"Dude, just divorce him. You deserve better."

That phone call was the final push I needed. Hearing it, again,
from a friend I wasn't particularly close to, produced a clearer
picture of my situation with Michael. There was nothing left
to hold on to with him.

When Michael got home from New York, I told him we
needed to talk. While Atticus napped upstairs, I sat at my kitchen
island and said, "I know you're with Carla. Please don't try to
deny it. Everyone knows. I don't hate you, but I want a divorce."

He looked down at his feet. "Okay. I'm sorry."

"I'm sorry I held on so long."

And with that, with little pomp and circumstance, we agreed to end our marriage.

I knew that Michael wouldn't follow through with trying to get custody of Atticus. By this point, I'd learned that he was all bark. He never would have spent the money on his own attorney, and I believe that in his heart he knew he couldn't provide for Atticus in the ways I could, in the ways I had.

I went upstairs to Atticus's room, put on a CD, and crawled in next to him on his toddler bed. His little sleeping body sensed my presence and curled into me, his tiny arm wrapping its way around my side.

The music drifted in the air as I shut my eyes—*and the pure light within you guide your way on.*

CHAPTER 26
Exit Music
2005–2008

After Michael and I separated, I'd naively thought that all of my dysfunctional relationship crap was behind me. I was off of drugs, had learned the ropes of functioning as an adult, was a mom. All of the old behavior, all of the old depression and anxiety and acting out should've been over and done. If only it had been that easy.

Drugs were decidedly in the rearview for me. I didn't struggle to stay clean. I'd left the twelve-step program I'd been involved with because there was a lot of emotional baggage there and it had become too much for me to deal with the ghosts of old me. The problem was the ghosts were part of me.

In January of 2006, Bea and I forged ahead with the clothing line and became friends with Ryan, the photographer of our first look book. Ryan was handsome—dark haired and a little scruffy in a Jake Gyllenhaal sort of way. He was five years younger than me and from the first day we met, I knew he'd be in my life for a very long time. What I felt for Ryan was intense but wasn't romantic love; I saw him more like a little brother or partner in crime. The most significant part of our relationship is that we didn't sleep together; we didn't muddy the waters with sex.

With Ryan, I learned how to have fun again—as an individual, separate from my identity as a mom. After Michael moved out, Ryan moved in and would be my roommate off and on for the next five years. Through Ryan, I met a whole new group of friends, some in LA and some in New York. Life felt light and free and full of possibilities.

Ellen, my best friend from high school, had reached out to me on Myspace and we rekindled our friendship. As Bea and I struggled to get our clothing line off the ground, Bea decided she didn't want to continue. Ellen became my new business partner. We got a showroom and started making sales, landing in boutiques and a high-end department store.

In the fall of 2006, I was ready to date again. I met a guy, another record producer, in New York, and we started seeing each other. Between the clothing line and my love life, I was flying back and forth every few weeks, Atticus staying with my mom and occasionally with Michael.

One of the friends I'd made through Ryan was Ralph, another photographer; they'd gone to art school together. Ralph was also five years younger than me—tall, fair, and handsome in a wholesome Midwest way, almost always wearing some variation of A.P.C. jeans, white T-shirt, flannel, and glasses. We hit it off right away. We talked to each other about our dating lives. And more and more, he was my last text of the day and my first text of the morning. By January of 2007, our light flirtation led to sex. I broke things off with the guy I'd been seeing, and Ralph and I started dating.

Dating was different now that I had Atticus. Ralph was great with kids, great with Atticus, but when we talked about our future, it scared the hell out of him. By summer, I planned to move to New York. The day I'd found a family to rent my house, he called me and told me he couldn't continue seeing me. He wasn't ready for the responsibilities of committing to me. I was blindsided. In the days that followed, I stopped eating, I threatened to kill myself. I had a meltdown at a pool party at Bea's house in front of many of my friends and in front of four-year-old Atticus.

When I flew to New York a couple of weeks later, I stayed with my friend Garett. I'd met him through Ryan as well. He was another photographer and had also gone to school with Ryan and Ralph. He'd been in LA when I had my pool party breakdown and was concerned about me seeing Ralph. We sat on the couch in his small Williamsburg apartment.

"So, I'm meeting Ralph for dinner," I said.

"Dude," he said, shaking his head, throwing his long, skinny legs up onto the coffee table. "I'm kind of worried about that, to be honest."

Garrett was friends with both of us but was not a fan of "us" as a couple. He could see the dysfunction long before anyone else could, or at least long before anyone else said.

"It's just dinner," I said.

But dinner led to spending the night, led to picking up my suitcase from Garrett's, led to talking, led to arguing, led to me acting like I'd lost my damn mind. And maybe I had.

"Hi," I said to Ralph's neighbor with a reluctant wave, holding my non-waving hand over my face, pretending to shield it from the late-afternoon sun but actually trying to hide my scratched, swollen face and puffy, red eyes.

I sat on the steep steps outside Ralph's apartment in Carroll Gardens, taking deep breaths and trying to center myself. I don't remember how the conversation had started or how the conversation had turned into an argument or how the conversation had turned into us breaking up, again.

What I do know is that I flew into a panic, into a fury, into the kind of emotional tornado that I couldn't control. I screamed that I wanted to die, I bashed my head into the white wall above his bed, I scratched at my face and slapped myself and threw myself on the ground and wailed.

Ralph, ever pragmatic, told me, then begged me to stop. Reminded me the neighbors could hear me; *they might call the police.* I walked to the bathroom and splashed my sore face with cold water and then stepped outside to take a breath. I felt embarrassed, no, humiliated. It had been over four years since I'd used drugs and yet I still struggled to gain control over my behavior. This was the first serious relationship I had without being on drugs at some point. Thirteen-year-old me was trying to be thirty-three-year-old me, and she didn't know how.

For the next couple of years, Ralph and I broke up and got together repeatedly. Sometimes I dated other people when we were apart. Sometimes I just fell to pieces. Sometimes I went numb.

Meanwhile, my clothing line business with Ellen fell apart. And I didn't handle that like an adult either. I avoided situations and made a mess, and we stopped speaking again for a while.

As my love life flip-flopped and my business went down the drain with the economy in 2008, I started working in production with Danica. I fell into periods of deep depression and anxiety. And I didn't talk about it. I didn't turn to drugs, but I did turn to spending money I didn't have, racking up credit card debt, and acting out—lashing out at friends, at Ralph, and occasionally at Atticus. I felt like I was failing in every area of my life.

That same year Bea and Dale split up. It was a shock to everyone, and I felt like I was losing my surrogate parents. My role models for a healthy relationship couldn't make it work. How could I ever manage it?

In early September of 2008, on a sweltering Saturday afternoon, I was prepping for a production job I was working with Danica. Five-year-old Atticus sat on a stool at the kitchen island, watching a *Fairly OddParents* cartoon while I was folding kitchen towels. Suddenly, I couldn't focus my eyes, the left side of my face scrunched up and froze, and I couldn't move my left arm.

Am I having a stroke? Please, God, don't let me be like The Diving Bell and the Butterfly.

"Mama, what's wrong?" asked Atticus.

"I just need to go lie down for a minute," I said.

I walked into the living room and lay down on a Persian rug in the entryway. The next thing I remember I was upstairs in my bedroom. I looked around and saw that I'd changed my sheets and folded towels. I didn't remember doing any of it. My phone was ringing.

"Hello?"

"Hi, honey."

It was Mom.

"Mom, I feel kind of weird," I said, walking downstairs.

I found Atticus in the kitchen, still watching cartoons. "Atticus, do you remember Mommy wasn't feeling well? I can't remember what happened."

"Your face was all funny," he said, scrunching his face up. "And you said you couldn't see."

"Mom, I think maybe I had a stroke."

Mom picked us up, and we drove to the ER of the hospital where my stepdad works. It was the same hospital where I'd detoxed on my first trip to rehab more than a decade earlier. They ran a whole battery of tests and referred me to a neurologist and cardiologist. It wasn't a stroke. It was a complex partial seizure. I'd lost time, about twenty minutes. But none of my tests showed any evidence of epilepsy.

Over the next two weeks, I had an EKG, an EEG, an MRI, and an ultrasound of my carotid artery. My carotid artery was just fine, but the technician found a large mass on my right thyroid. A few days later I had another ultrasound and a needle biopsy. It was not cancerous, but it was large—about the size of a golf ball—and the doctors didn't want to leave it there as it would likely cause problems with swallowing and turn cancerous at some point.

On Halloween 2008, I had surgery to remove my right thyroid and two right parathyroids. We never found out what caused the seizure and I never had one again. The woo-woo part of me thinks it was the universe's way of getting that mass out of my body. Maybe if it had been left there, I would have ended up with cancer or tracheal issues. The health scare additionally brought me back to practicing Kundalini yoga and meditation. It was a reminder that I needed to work on my spiritual wellness again. I'd lost track of it among relationship problems and letting go of my business.

In June of 2009, Ralph and I broke up yet again, days before Atticus and I left for a three-week vacation in Italy with Dad; my stepmom, Stacy; Anya; and my stepsister, Laura. I was severely depressed on the trip, despite the epic beauty of Tuscany. I sent angry text messages to Ralph, who was in France working. By day we explored Montepulciano and Rome and Florence and Siena and Venice and Abruzzo and Luca. At night, I cried myself to sleep.

Ryan was in New York working, staying at Ralph's new apartment in Williamsburg while he was in France. I decided to spend some time in New York before going home. It was a special kind of torture sleeping in Ralph's bed while he was gone, and I was trying to get over him. One afternoon, while Atticus spent time with Michael, who was upstate with his girlfriend, Ryan and two other friends and I drove out to Storm King—the spectacular outdoor sculpture garden about an hour from the city.

Ryan and I lay in the grass staring up at a giant red Calder sculpture; I turned to him and said, "I feel so lost. I feel like I could just float away and it would be like I was never here at all."

He turned his head and looked at me, narrowing his eyes. "You just need to find the thing that makes you want to get up in the morning, the thing that makes you feel alive. Not a person, but a calling."

"Oh, is that all," I said and we both laughed.

The next morning, Ryan flew back to Los Angeles, and Mary, who was now living in Rhode Island, drove into the city to meet up with me. As I waited for Mary, I got a call from Michael. He and his girlfriend had gotten in a fight. She'd kicked Michael and Atticus out of her house upstate, and they were taking the train back to New York City. Mary and I met them at Grand Central Station and also met up with Ethan, a guy Mary had been dating who lived in Brooklyn.

We had a very New York day; we did so much walking. We had brunch at Pastis, Michael, too. The conversation between us all cheered me up. Ethan was smart and funny and a writer. *He's so lucky*, I thought. *I wish I could do that.* We walked along the High Line and through Chelsea. We talked about life and work and relationships.

"I don't know what I want to be when I grow up," I said.

"I don't either," said Michael, laughing.

"You should write," said Ethan.

"What?"

"You should write. The way you tell stories and talk about life... They would make great essays."

"I haven't written in a long time."

I thought about the years of writing in journals. *But that's not real writing.* Still, his words got inside me, they entered my bloodstream and made music so loud I couldn't ignore them.

You should write.

CHAPTER 27
Home
2009–2016

When I got back to Ralph's empty apartment, Ethan's words continued to echo in my head. *You should write.* I put Atticus to bed and opened up my laptop. I created a Blogspot account and set up my blog—*Rarely Wrong Erin.* I named it this after an inside joke between me and Bea. It was her nickname for me, because people were always asking me for relationship advice. That, or the name of the actress who played Natalie on *The Facts of Life*—Mindy Cohn.

The next day, Michael picked up Atticus, and I went by myself to The Metropolitan Museum of Art. I took a photo of one of the Polish writer Stanisław Witkiewicz's photographs. I'd been obsessed with him in high school. Back at Ralph's apartment that night, after I'd packed our suitcases and put Atticus to bed, I wrote my first blog post and included the picture I'd taken. Then I started googling writing programs. Two hours deep into my search, I found that I could take online writing classes at The New School. I signed up for a creative nonfiction class that started a few weeks later.

Back in Los Angeles, I began blogging daily and writing morning pages, allowing my head to spill onto the page, to unload and find truth and meaning. That fall, in my first writing class in many years, my teacher invited me to meet her at a writing conference in New York. In October, I did just that. I worked on a piece about my first trip to rehab. My teacher, Lisa, made me believe in my writing, made me think I was capable of telling my story and helping others. It was when I first thought that maybe, one day, I would write a memoir.

Shortly after I'd started the blog, Bea listened to me give advice to another friend over dinner. Afterward, she said, "You should start an advice section of the blog. You're so good at this."

"Yeah, I'm good at it because I've made all the mistakes."

"That's your tagline!" she said.

And that's just what I did. Ask Erin was born. "She's made all the mistakes, so you don't have to… Ask Erin is an advice column, in which Erin answers your burning questions about anything at all." My little blog started to pick up steam, and I received questions from friends and strangers alike.

That fall, Ralph and I got back together, but things were different. I had found a calling—an identity and purpose outside mother or daughter or broken ex-junkie. The more I wrote, the more I felt sure of who I was. I continued taking writing courses and finally finished my undergraduate degree.

By March of 2011, Ralph and I were at another standstill. One night, during a tense phone call, I told Ralph I wanted a break. I needed to figure out what I wanted, and he needed to do the same. I went into Ryan's room and flopped down on his bed.

"I don't know what to do," I said. "I love him, but I feel like we've been going in circles for so long."

"You have been. You know I love the guy, but you're not really right for each other."

"Well, I just told him I wanted a break…"

286 ERIN KHAR

Ryan went to his desk and grabbed a notebook and pen. "We're making a list."

"A list?"

"Yes. A list of all the qualities you want in a partner."

Reluctantly, I did, putting aside my feelings of how hokey this was. I wanted someone who made me feel wanted, who loved me, who was funny and smart, who wanted marriage and possibly more kids, someone who challenged me but I could rely on, someone who wouldn't pull the rug out from under me.

I called Bea to see what she was doing. Cliff, a guy I'd dated during one of my breakups with Ralph and was still friends with, was coming to her apartment for dinner and drinks and to get advice about T-shirt manufacturing, as Bea was still working in the garment industry. She invited me to come, too.

I was feeling down and was grateful for the company. Cliff showed up with his friend and new roommate, Seth. I'd met Seth once, in passing, through Cliff. I didn't think much of him, except as *that friend of Cliff's*. But as we ate Indian food and talked and laughed at Bea's kitchen table, I realized how funny he was. He was Jewish, from New Jersey, and had a dry, sharp wit. And he was cute—light brown hair and long eyelashes and soft lips. He reminded me of Ryan Gosling with glasses. Toward the end of the night, he made a joke with the punch line "Penny Marshall," and it was like someone had struck me with Cupid's arrow. *He had me at* Penny Marshall.

Cliff, Seth, Bea, and I started spending more time together. I could feel myself falling for Seth. *But he's too young. He's seven years younger than me. I am done with younger guys.* Besides, Seth was dating someone. There was also the Cliff factor. I could sense that even though he was seeing someone and really liked her, he was still a little possessive when it came to me. *No, this is just not gonna happen.*

One night, I'd made dinner for all of us at my house. We had been swapping relationship stories. Arguably, mine were the most *colorful*. Seth laughed, took off his glasses, shook his head, and said, "Wow. You are my worst nightmare."

"What?" I asked, feeling hot around my neck.

"No, it's good information to have. I would *never* date someone like you."

"You don't even know me," I said, incensed. "You're going to sit there and judge me because I told you some outlandish stories from the past?"

We went back and forth like this. Cliff and Bea left the dining room and started cleaning up. Later, I sent Bea a text: What an asshole. Who does that guy think he is?

She answered back: Um, you guys are totally gonna get together.

I replied: Fuck that guy.

Less than two weeks later, we slept together. And we started spending every day together. He ended things with the girl he'd been seeing, and I ended things with Ralph once and for all. I immediately broke all the sensible relationship rules in getting together with Seth—we had sex immediately, I had dovetailed from the end of one relationship right into this one—but it all felt right; it felt different.

Seth brought strength and stability to our relationship. He made me feel calm, secure, and for a while, things sailed along without drama. He was wonderful with Atticus. He didn't try to be his best friend or step in as an instant parent. He was an adult; he modeled healthy behavior. Atticus trusted him; I could see that.

But as we got closer, I began acting out—starting fights, telling him we should break up because it wasn't going to work out anyway, accusing him of not loving me. Once again, as far as I had come, I was backsliding into old behaviors.

About six months into our relationship, we sat at dinner, where I'd launched into another round of *let me see how far I can push him*. The self-destructive part of me wanted him to break up with me, to prove to myself I was indeed unlovable and not worthy of someone's affection.

Rather than play my game, Seth took my hands in his and said, "Erin, I love you. I see a future with you. But if you don't do something to address this sabotaging behavior, our relationship is doomed."

I looked at him, this man I loved, as he said what I knew was true. I was sabotaging things. And I didn't know how to stop myself. But I heard him.

"You're right. I know I'm doing it, but I don't know how to stop. I promise, I'm going to get help."

Unlike the many promises to get help I'd made in previous relationships, this time I meant it. I wanted that future with Seth. I went back to therapy and went back on Wellbutrin, the medication that had worked well for me in the past, the one I probably should have stayed on. Over the years, with therapists and psychiatrists and rehab, I'd dipped my toes in facing my issues with men and intimacy, but I never jumped in. I had to jump in, or I was going to lose the healthiest relationship and best partner I'd ever had.

In 2013, Atticus and I moved to New York City, where Seth's career had brought him. Atticus and I converted to Judaism, which surprisingly was at Atticus's urging. In Judaism we both found a spiritual center, one I didn't know was possible in organized religion. In August of 2014, Seth and I married. My writing career progressed, and Seth and I began trying to have a second child. My life had arrived at a safe harbor, a place I'd never thought possible.

As Atticus's thirteenth birthday loomed, I thought back to the question he'd asked me nine months earlier about why people took drugs.

I knocked on Atticus's door and pushed it slightly open. "Atticus, honey, can I come in?"

"Mom, you're supposed to wait for me to answer before you push the door open," he said, not taking his eyes off the TV screen, Xbox controller in hand.

I smiled. "I know. Hey, I want to talk to you for a minute."

"Now?"

"Well, yeah."

He rolled his eyes and spoke into his headset. "Hey, I gotta go talk to my mom. Be right back."

He shut off the TV and I sat on his bed, taking a deep breath.

"You remember a while back, you asked me if I ever did drugs?"

"Yeah."

"Well, I didn't really answer your question then and I feel like I need to."

"Okay."

"You know, when I was a kid, younger than you, I started feeling really sad. And I didn't know what to do with those feelings. I didn't tell my parents how I was feeling. I felt like I wanted to hurt myself and even felt sometimes like I wanted to die."

He sat up, suddenly tuned in to the weight of what I was saying, and asked, "Why were you so sad?"

I took another deep breath and exhaled. "Well, part of it is that my brain works a little differently than most people's. I have depression and I didn't understand that when I was a kid. It scared me. And then there were things that happened when I was a kid that were traumatic for me, and I didn't talk about it with anyone."

"I'm sorry, Mom."

I felt a lump in my throat but continued, "I didn't know what to do with all those feelings. I made some really bad decisions. And one of those bad decisions is that I started using drugs."

"You did?" he asked, his eyes wide.

"I did."

"Pot?"

"No. I used a lot of things, but mostly heroin."

"Heroin? Like *Pulp Fiction*?"

"Yeah."

"Whoa...when you were a kid?"

"I was really young, only a little bit older than you."

"Does Seth know?"

"Yeah, Seth knows."

"Do Mom and Bompa know?" he asked, using his names for my parents.

"Yeah, they know. They didn't know until I was in my twenties."

"You used drugs that whole time?"

"Not all the time, but yeah, I struggled with drugs for a long time, until I was pregnant with you."

"Do you use drugs now?"

"No. I haven't used drugs since before you were born."

We sat in silence for a moment. I looked out the window, past the fire escape outside, looking at the shadows in the window across the courtyard. A mother and young child were at the window chatting. Our little poodle mix, Pretty Lady, barked from the living room at phantom noises in the hallway outside. Atticus named her when he was five. (You can imagine the looks you get calling "Pretty Lady" down the streets of New York.)

"Pretty, be quiet!" yelled Atticus.

"So, the reason I'm telling you this, the reason I felt like it was important... Well, it's a couple of reasons actually. First of all, you know I write. And a lot of what I write is read by people online. I didn't want you to find things out online that I hadn't told you. And the other reason is that I was only a couple of months older than you when I first tried drugs. I want you to know that while I hope you don't make those kinds of choices, that if you do, you can come to me. Even if I am sad or disappointed, I will never judge you, and I will always love you.

I wish I had asked for help when I was a teenager. The good thing is that now I don't feel that way. I'm not perfect. I still make mistakes. But I know how to take care of myself, I know how to ask for help, and I take medication for my depression."

Atticus's big golden-brown eyes were glassy and he leaned forward and put his arms around me, a show of affection that was becoming less frequent as he got older. He put his head on my shoulder and said, "Mom, I'm so sorry you had to go through all that. I'm glad you're okay."

The lump in my throat bloomed and I let the tears come. "Thank you, honey. I love you so much."

"I love you, too, Mom."

The conversation I'd been afraid to have felt like grace. In the years since our conversation, as Atticus has grown and changed in his teenage years, he's asked me more questions, and I've answered honestly, without being overly graphic. It's vital we have these conversations with our kids. Teenagers need to know that they can survive even their greatest mistakes.

Watching Atticus grow up has created a mirror for me. When he turned thirteen, I thought about me at thirteen—hiding and yet so desperate to be seen. I thought I was grown-up, taking control over a life that felt out of control by using heroin. I was a little girl. Through motherhood, I have grown to have empathy for young Erin, to mother her, too. As much as I've beat myself up over the years for the many poor decisions I made, I also see them now as survival. I was a lost and scared child, trying to survive.

My empathy has also grown toward my parents. They made some mistakes, like I have with Atticus. But they never turned their backs on me. They never stopped loving me. Even when I was at my worst. Even when I lied to them and manipulated them and stole from them. They remained steadfast in my life. When I asked for help, they helped me. They have seen some of the darkest parts of me and they're still here. I am filled with gratitude for that.

Becoming a mother rebuilt my relationship with my own mom. I understand her in ways I couldn't before. She has stood by me. We have been able to talk about the past, about my childhood, with transparency and openness. She has validated my experiences and what I felt. And she has continued to mother her adult daughter. Because I still needed it. I still needed her.

As I've recovered, I've rebuilt and repaired my relationships with the people who loved me when I couldn't love myself. Lila and Diana and Polly are all in my life. We've recovered, together; we've become mothers and wives and have careers. I've maintained friendships with most of my exes. I've tried to make amends to whomever I could, however I could. And Michael and I have managed to maintain a cordial relationship as Atticus's parents.

The most important healing I've done is with the relationship I have with myself. All that time, all those years, I was looking for someone or something to save me—my parents, money, grades, accomplishments, drugs, sex, love.

But it was me all along.

The only one who could save me was me. Nora Ephron once said, "Above all, be the heroine of your own life…"

I can finally say that I am.

I am in awe of the circular nature of life. I'm amazed at the journey it took to get me here. And I'm so happy to be alive.

CHAPTER 28
After All

I have often compared my years spent in active addiction to being in a room on fire. With each passing year, with each line I crossed that I'd said I wouldn't, those flames got bigger, those flames got closer. And I couldn't figure a way out of the room. Every exit I approached was too thick with smoke and fire to get through. The last time I detoxed—when I was pregnant with Atticus—I knew that I couldn't stay in that room any longer, that staying in that room would kill us both. I made a decision to walk through the flames and fortunately made it out. I didn't know until I'd walked right through that it had been the solution all long.

As I believe is true with most compulsions, for opiate addicts, the only way out is through—through the pain and the shame and the trauma, through facing the very things we ran from when we turned to drugs. That is the beginning.

Escaping addiction, and it truly does feel like an escape, requires protective layers of aftercare. I have been incredibly fortunate to have access to the support I've needed. We don't have a system in place that makes it simple or easy for people to get help or support. There are financial, social, and racial barriers to getting help. If we are going to see a real downshift in the opiate crisis, support is what is needed—not just from peers and family members, but also the medical community and government.

Mental illness is a large part of my story. Crushing depression was a constant, looming companion throughout my life. I've joked that my depression and addiction were in a codependent relationship. It's true. They fed off each other. It should come as no surprise that people with mental health issues are more than three times more likely to use opiates.[3] We can't begin to address the opiate crisis in earnest without treating underlying mental health issues.

I have stayed on medication since 2012, and it has transformed my life. I accepted that my brain works differently and needs chemical help to function well. Certainly, I'm not happy all the time, but in general, I am. I don't have the extreme highs and lows; I don't act out in destructive ways; I can mostly regulate my emotions. And with time and therapy and further spiritual searching, I have healed and continue to heal.

I have learned how to stay.

I have learned how to sit in discomfort and grief. I have learned how to be in a relationship, a partnership. I have learned how to stop looking for an exit.

After Seth and I married, we started trying for a second child. In 2017, after two years, four miscarriages, and a devastating second-trimester loss, we welcomed a second child, Franklin, to our family. I got through those two years with the tools I've learned. Having gone through sexual abuse, rape, heroin addiction, and mental illness—and experiencing the PTSD of all of it—I had to learn how to make it through extreme pain without

---

3   Matthew A. Davis, Lewei A. Lin, Haiyin Liu, and Brian D. Sites, "Prescription Opioid Use among Adults with Mental Health Disorders in the United States," *Journal of the American Board of Family Medicine* 30, no. 4 (July 2017): 407–417, https://doi.org/10.3122/jabfm.2017.04.170112.

destroying my life. I had to grow spiritually and mentally and emotionally. That growth has made me capable of facing life in a way I didn't think I could.

Over the past few years, I have published essays about my addiction and spoken publicly about my past with unflinching honesty. I can look at my past today without a shred of shame. I am not made of the mistakes I made; I am made of how I got up again after I made them. I am made of speaking the truth, of doing my best, of being willing to fail still and grow and learn.

I moved my advice column to *Ravishly* in 2015, where it has grown exponentially. Every month, hundreds of people write to me asking for advice. They ask me if they should stay in dysfunctional relationships, if they should try polyamory, if I think they have a drug problem. They ask me how to handle overbearing in-laws, how to set a boundary, how to get through the pain of heartbreak or loss of a child. People come to me because they need someone else to say out loud what they already know. They come to me because they're lost. They come to me because they know I might have been through it, too.

I have the privilege of sharing my experience, strength, and hope from all those thousands of mistakes I made.

Someone once asked me, about my writing, "Don't you want to leave all that mess behind you?"

When we write the truth, when we write about our experiences, we reflect back what it means to be a human being. And that reflection creates connection. I write what I know, what I've learned, and about the road that got me from there to here. We turn to art and make art to feel less alone, to stir something, to think, to breathe, to dream, to recover. I have said this before, and it remains true for me—I have no desire to run from my past, to not look back to "all that mess." That mess is part of me, that mess has allowed me to live and be here today. I hope that by sharing my story with you, I make you feel less alone.

My other great hope is that this book helps to alleviate the stigma around opiate addiction. I hope that you can look at those who struggle with opiate addiction with renewed compassion and empathy. If you're the one struggling with addiction, I hope you reach out for help. I hope you know it's possible. I hope you know you are worthwhile and meant to be here.

My life today is unrecognizable from what it once was. At eight, at thirteen, at twenty-three, at twenty-six, at twenty-nine, I never would have believed the peace and happiness I found was possible. I didn't think I could let go of the shame. I didn't think I could tell the truth. I didn't think I could forgive myself or not see myself as a monster. For so many years, I didn't think I'd make it out of addiction and depression alive. I was certain that I'd meet my end in overdose or by suicide.

But here I am.

This book is for the ones who didn't make it. This book is for the ones who survived. This book is for the ones who are still struggling. I see you. I believe in you.

I love you.

★ ★ ★ ★ ★

ACKNOWLEDGMENTS

Pieces of this memoir, in different forms, have appeared in *Best New Writing 2012*, *Mr. Beller's Neighborhood*, and *Haunted Waters Press: From the Depths*.

Huge thanks to my phenomenal agents, Jeff Kleinman and Erin Harris of Folio Literary Management, for believing in me, championing me, and making this book happen.

Thank you to my editor, Laura Brown, for sharing a vision with me, for making this book infinitely better because of her edits, for being patient with my many, many em dashes, and for being a guiding light, a mentor, and a friend. Thanks to the many folks at Park Row Books for believing in this book and making the publishing process a dream come true. I knew from our first meeting that Park Row was home. Thank you, Erika Imranyi, editorial director of Park Row; Margaret Marbury, VP Trade; Loriana Sacilotto, executive VP Editorial; Emer Flounders, publicity director; Roxanne Jones, publicity director; Heather Foy, VP of Sales; Linette Kim, library marketing manager; Randy Chan, senior marketing manager; Amy Jones, senior director of marketing; Marketing Director Rachel Haller; copy editor Chris Wolfgang.

I am forever indebted to my writing community—Eric Wybenga for telling me to write; Lisa Freedman for making me believe I could write a whole book; Lauren Jonik for reading the earliest of pages; Sue Shapiro for being so generous with your time and advice; Kimberlee Auerbach Berlin for helping me find the narrative; Jen McLellan for your pep talks; Emily Maloney for your daily check-ins; Marnie Goodfriend, Leslie Kendall Dye, and all my WWJs for listening to me vent, cry, laugh, and work my way through the publishing process; Lauren DePino for your continuous encouragement and friendship; Amy Klein, Naomi Rand, Patricia Grisafi, and Keren Blankfeld for notes and reassurance and cheering me on through writing the damn thing; Lilly Dancyger and Lisa Marie Basile for being incredible editors and friends; and Jennifer Pastiloff, Reema Zaman, and Stephanie Land for your love, kindness, and support.

Thank you to Lidia Yuknavitch for writing the introduction and for inspiring me, teaching me, for showing me love, and for creating Corporeal Writing, where some of this book took shape.

To my *Ravishly* family—past and present—thank you for being my sisters and friends, Jenni Berrett for your tarot card readings, and Joni Edelman, thank you for everything—for the job and the column space and the texts and the love.

Thank you to the friends and guides whose kindnesses they may not even remember but which I will never forget, for you changed my life—Ana Gulde, Andre Neyrey, Andrew Clark, Barrie Fuller, Bob Forrest, Cali Thornhill DeWitt, Camille Garmendia, Cheyann Benedict, Craig Brewer, Davey Faragher, Diane Davis, Dr. Gregory, Dr. Drew Pinsky, Dr. Pylko, Emily Wroe, Eric Erlandson, Eric Niles, Franck Nataf, Hallie Goodman, Hunter Shepherd, Jennifer Krasinski, Jessica Brodkin, Jimmy Boyle, Jordan Granger, Julie Shaub, Justin Hollar, Kathleen Burke,

Kristi Matamoros, Larry Schemel, Leslie Wolf, Lisa Simmons, Marco Badenchini, Martin Klingman, Michelle Albuquerque, Mike Semple, Norman Reedus, Patty DiMaria, Patty Schemel, Peter Johansen, Phillip Hutson, Rebecca Rose Perkins, Rosemary Fuller, Sonya Farrell, Sweet P, Tania Saylor, Truly Rain, Wendy Maring, and many, many more.

Thank you to the beautiful humans who loved me when I couldn't love myself—Ben Grieme, Blackie Rowan, Bonnie Faragher, Brian Smith, Dawnne Aubert, Eric Boyles, Erica Paige, Erin Ballew, Gregoire Valot, Joy Sherrick, K, Lara Vanian-Green, Melinda Mara, Nick Cooper, Patricia Castaneda, Patrick Paeper, RJ Shaughnessy, Roya Parivar, and Scott Addison.

Infinite thanks to my family who've loved me and accepted me, despite my missteps—my cousin K and aunt D for always being there; my stepparents, who I am so lucky to have in my life; my sister and stepsiblings, who have given me the family I didn't know I needed; and my in-laws, who welcomed Atticus and me with open arms.

Thank you to my parents, who continued to love me even when I made it nearly impossible.

Thank you, Seth. You taught me how to stay. I love you.

Thank you, Franklin, our rainbow baby—you made our family complete.

And thank you, Atticus—you saved my life and taught me how to love.